# REWIRING

# TINNITUS

## HOW I FINALLY FOUND RELIEF FROM
## THE RINGING IN MY EARS

# GLENN SCHWEITZER

# Disclaimer

This book contains only the opinions and ideas of its author who is neither a doctor nor a medical professional. It is in no way intended as a substitute for the advice of medical professionals. The reader should consult a medical professional before adopting any of the suggestions in this book and in all matters relating to his/her health, particularly with respect to any medications, supplements, and symptoms that may require diagnosis or medical attention.

Cover design by *Popdesign*☼

ISBN-13: 978-1540483188
ISBN-10: 1540483185

For my parents,

Paul and Randi Schweitzer,

Who listen to me go on and on about my latest obsessions, no matter how enthusiastic I am. Who showed me how to face adversity with a smile on my face. Who raised a difficult kid, but never gave up on me. Who offer encouragement when I'm down, support when I need it most, and a helping hand when it all falls apart. Their love shaped me into the man I am today.

# Contents

# Acknowledgements

Writing this book was a lonely endeavor, but it took a village to get it done. I want to take a moment to thank all the people who helped me turn this book into something I'm proud of.

First and foremost, I want to give a special thanks to my editor, Philippa Thomson. Her experience, professionalism, and knowledge was invaluable. She took my words and made them shine.

I want to thank my wife, Megan. She has stuck by my side, supporting me through every hardship I've faced with my health. She read through every draft, editing out my clutter and offering valuable feedback. Thousands of commas died at her hands.

I also want to thank my grandmother, Ellie, who took the time to edit my early drafts, helping me shape my words into something that made sense. She's one of the few people in my family that understands how horrible tinnitus can be.

I want to thank all the other people who read the first draft of my manuscript and gave me feedback. Your ideas and suggestions were so important to me.

And finally, I want to give a special heartfelt thanks to my readers. Without your love and support, I would never have taken on a project like this. I'm inspired every day by your comments, stories, messages and feedback. You mean the world to me!

# **Introduction**

The sudden noise sent a shockwave through my brain and jolted me out of my TV trance.

It sounded like sirens, several of them, blaring over a gust of wind, and caused a terrible pressure to build in my ears.

I could feel my heart pounding in my chest. My eyes darted around the room, frantically searching my small apartment for the source of the sound. My roommate was still sleeping, my girlfriend too, and my phone was on silent.

It wasn't the fire alarm either. I was alone with the TV.

Maybe it was coming from outside? I stumbled over to the sliding glass door and went out into my screened-in patio. But nothing seemed out of the ordinary. It was almost 1 am and the air was humid and stagnant. Everything was calm.

I started to panic. My mind was racing, desperately trying to make sense of the situation. Maybe I was hallucinating somehow? I felt dizzy, could it be food poisoning? I had no idea. I was grasping at straws.

Back inside, I collapsed on the couch. The sound had been blasting for several minutes now. I couldn't even hear myself think. Maybe I was losing my mind.

But then something clicked into place. I suddenly knew with absolute certainty that there was no noise, at least not outside my head. I wasn't hallucinating either, not in the traditional sense at any rate.

A word had quietly floated up from the depths of my subconscious mind and was now flashing across my awareness like a neon sign: tinnitus.

My breathing started to slow down, at least a little.

The noise was staggering, but I knew its name, and for the time being that was enough. I had never experienced anything like it before, but at the same time, it wasn't exactly new either.

You see, I've had ringing in my ears for as long as I can remember; it had just never been this loud or this violent.

I didn't know it at the time, but everything in my

life was about to change. The ground was shifting under my feet, and I wasn't prepared.

The unfortunate reality is that every day hundreds of millions of people around the world are endlessly tormented by noises that no one else can hear. For some, it's high pitched tones, whistles, beeps or clicks. For others, it's chirps, whooshing or buzzing noises, like the sound of a jet engine.

When you live with tinnitus, the medical term for ringing in the ears, the sound never stops, and it can quickly turn life into a living nightmare.

I've had tinnitus for a long time, but it hasn't always bothered me. In fact, when I was younger it never even occurred to me that other people couldn't hear the high-pitched sound that I could hear when it was quiet. I thought it was normal.

But five years ago, as I sat on the couch watching Seinfeld re-runs late one night, things suddenly got a whole lot worse.

At the time, I was four months away from being diagnosed with a somewhat rare, incurable inner ear disorder called Meniere's disease. It's a particularly nasty condition that causes vertigo, tinnitus, hearing loss and a feeling of pressure in the ears.

My panicked experience with the sound of sirens was but a small taste of things to come. Meniere's disease changed everything for me. After my diagnosis, my tinnitus was no longer the quiet, high pitched tone that I was used to. It became much louder, and was layered with lower pitched tones and a constant whooshing sound that made it hard to fall asleep, and even harder to focus. The noise steadily added to the already high levels of anxiety that I was experiencing as a result of my diagnosis. The sound tormented me, day and night.

But that was then. Fast forward a few years, and I'm happy to report that my tinnitus no longer bothers me at all. Completely by accident, I stumbled onto techniques that radically rewired my emotional, psychological, and physical response to the sound. Almost overnight, it stopped bothering me.

And I know that I'm not alone. One way or another, many people do learn to live comfortably with tinnitus. And that's a good thing because it's a big problem.

According to the Center for Disease Control, nearly 50 million people suffer from tinnitus in the United States alone. It's also the most prevalent disability among our nation's veterans, even outranking post-traumatic stress disorder (PTSD). Worldwide, the number of sufferers is estimated to be close to 600 million. As I said, it's a big problem.

If you suffer from tinnitus, I want you to know right now that there is so much hope. No matter how severe it is, or how bad things may seem, you can learn to live with your tinnitus too.

I will show you the way. I'll teach you everything I've learned on my successful journey with tinnitus. I will give you all the tools and techniques that finally brought me relief, and gave me back my quality of life. Because you deserve to have peace and a life of happiness, too.

This book is divided into three sections, each one designed to bring you a step closer toward this goal. The first section will give you a detailed understanding of tinnitus. I will start with my personal story, detailing my struggles and ultimate triumph over the noise. I will explain how hearing works and how we process sound. You will understand exactly what tinnitus is, and the underlying conditions that can cause it. You will also learn how tinnitus can become so problematic and what you can do to address the fundamental issues that may be preventing you from experiencing relief.

In the second section, I will walk you through my unique approach to managing tinnitus step by step. You will learn to perform simple exercises that, over a short period of time, can radically alter the way you are affected by your tinnitus. I will show you how to use all of the tools and techniques that you need for success. You will walk away with a clear understanding of what it takes to improve.

And finally, in the third section, I will show you how to live your best life with tinnitus. I will teach you how to track your health and lifestyle to identify your triggers, the avoidable factors that can exacerbate your tinnitus. I will teach you how to protect your ears and your hearing to prevent your tinnitus from getting worse. You'll learn to manage your stress levels, while improving your overall health. I will show you how to sleep more soundly and fall asleep faster. And finally, I will leave you with a clear plan of action, one that can quickly produce results.

There may not be a cure for tinnitus, but there is a way forward. You can learn to live in harmony with the sound. It may not go away, but it will stop bothering you, and at the end of the day that's just as good.

Let's dive in.

# Part 1: Understanding Tinnitus

# Chapter 1
# **My Story**

"When the unthinkable happens, the lighthouse is hope. Once we choose hope, everything is possible."
- Christopher Reeve, actor

There is a distinct possibility that I was born with tinnitus, though it's hard to say for sure. What I do know is that I can't remember a time without it. For me, silence is nothing more than a lost memory. And while I can't say for certain when the ringing started, I do remember the first time it became a problem. I was only 13 years old.

For most of my young life the ringing was constant, but always quiet, and it never really bothered me. I thought it was normal. It wasn't until I overheard my father and grandmother talking about their tinnitus that I knew otherwise. I had always just assumed everyone could hear it. I remember saying, "Hey wait, I have that too! That's not normal?" At the time, though, it didn't matter. It was just a part of me that I lived with, and all I'd ever known.

That changed in seventh grade, when at 13 years old, several of my friends had Bar and Bat Mitzvahs. For the uninitiated, it's a Jewish ceremony that signifies one's passage into adulthood, and after the ceremony there's usually a party. They're a lot of fun, but also very loud, which I didn't know would be a problem.

At some point in their lives, most people will temporarily hear ringing in their ears and experience mild hearing loss, if only for a short period of time, after prolonged exposure to loud noise. It typically only lasts for a few hours - a day or two at most. If you've ever been to a loud concert, you probably know what I mean. But what most people don't know is that every time this happens, they are damaging their hearing. And if they have tinnitus, it can make it much, much worse.

I remember having a great time at my first Bar Mitzvah party. I drank soda, ate cake, and hung out with my friends. The band played good music, and everyone was happy. It wasn't until the car ride home that I noticed something was wrong.

It felt like there was cotton in my ears, and the ringing was much louder than normal. It was hard to hear the radio. I asked my parents, who had also attended the party, if their ears were ringing too. They both said yes and explained it was something that could happen when the music was too loud. I didn't really understand what they meant, but later that night I couldn't fall asleep. The ringing was deafening and it kept me awake for hours. I wanted it to stop so badly, but nothing would make it go away. Covering my ears only made it worse. I eventually fell asleep, but not before I tossed and turned for half the night.

When I woke the next morning, the ringing still wasn't back to its normal volume. It was better than it had been the night before, but I still felt uncomfortable. Another 12 hours passed before it quieted back down.

I guess it was good that at 13 I was still invincible. I was too young, too hyper, too curious for my tinnitus to ever really be a problem. But, as time passed, every loud party and concert would cause the whole cycle to repeat itself: mild hearing loss, loud ringing, tossing and turning in bed, then a slow return to normal. I had no idea that I was damaging my hearing, that I was making my tinnitus worse.

When I was in high school, the local rock station hosted a massive, multi-day, music festival at RFK Stadium. (It's where the Washington Redskins used to play.) My friends and I would always go to watch our favorite bands. I loved it. But in my junior year, I stood too close to the speakers during several of the performances.

Driving home afterward was rough. My ears felt destroyed, and for the next three days my hearing was terrible. Everything sounded as though it was being filtered through a tin can. I know that I did serious damage to my hearing that day. I wish I'd known better.

## Meniere's Disease

It wasn't until much later that tinnitus became a truly disruptive force in my life.

I was in my senior year of college at Florida Atlantic University as a Business and IT major. I had a steady girlfriend, good grades, and great friends. Life was going well, and more importantly I was happy. Happier than I had been in a long time. And when the rug was finally pulled out from under me, I had a long way to fall.

Most people will never know what it's like to stare down the barrel of a complex medical diagnosis.

That's not to say they'll never get sick - they probably will. And it might be terrible. But in most cases, it will at least be easy to comprehend. The implications will be clear, the treatment options will be explained, and the doctor will be knowledgeable. They will most likely know what to do next.

But for the unlucky few who are diagnosed with a complicated, rare disease, there are no certainties. There is little understanding. There is pain, confusion, and despair.

I was about to learn this firsthand.

When I found myself dizzy on the couch with my tinnitus sirens blaring, it was only the beginning: the earliest stages of Meniere's disease, a chronic illness with no known cause or cure. The symptoms include violent attacks of rotational vertigo, as well as progressive hearing loss, a feeling of fullness and pressure in the ears, and tinnitus. But I didn't know any of this at the time. I suffered without any kind of understanding for months, getting worse every single day.

When you've never experienced vertigo before, it's absolutely terrifying, especially when you don't know what's going on or why it's happening. It completely incapacitates you, often for hours on end. Your body, thinking it's been poisoned, makes you feel nauseous, so you start throwing up. But it offers no relief because there is no poison. The room just keeps spinning, and it becomes impossible to focus your eyes or stand up. It's also unpredictable. You hope it happens when you're somewhere safe, but that's not always the case. Many people get injured falling to the ground, or worse, hitting their head as the spinning starts. When it's over, you're left feeling cognitively impaired and thoroughly exhausted.

My first vertigo attack happened several weeks after my incident on the couch with tinnitus. I was in the middle of a lecture at school, an evening class held in one of the computer labs on campus. We were learning to build and manage computer databases.

On my walk over, I grabbed a bag of Chex-Mix from the food stand in the lobby. I was usually hungry by the time this class rolled around, and almost always bought something to eat while I worked on the computer.

But this time, shortly after I finished eating, my tinnitus suddenly exploded in volume again, and I felt a sharp pressure in my right ear. It all happened fast. Before I could even process what was going on, the room started spinning like I was on a tilt-a-whirl. I somehow managed to keep the food down, but I was extremely nauseous the entire time. In hindsight, it was only a minor attack, triggered by the high sodium content of the Chex-Mix, but even small attacks can be terrifying. My shirt was soaked with sweat, and I couldn't focus my eyes. I held on to the desk as the minutes ticked by, but there was still almost an hour to go.

I have no idea how I made it through the rest of the

class. After a certain point everything became a blur. I was scared. I had no answers and nothing made sense. I'm not even sure how I made the drive home. I'm lucky to be alive, and lucky that I didn't hurt anyone else.

But at the time, I was still firmly set in denial. As scared as I was, deep down I was more afraid to go to the doctor. I wasn't ready to let the problem become real. After all, this symptom was new and it had only happened once. I was sure that I would get better. But that's not what happened. Over the following months, things continued to get worse. The attacks started to happen more frequently, and in between attacks I felt dizzy most of the time. Driving became challenging and dangerous. I was also tired most of the time, and my tinnitus kept getting louder. The constant noise made it hard for me to fall asleep, and the lack of rest was making all of my symptoms worse. The ringing also made it difficult to focus at school, and my grades started to slip. But I pressed on in denial, always ready with an excuse, as if it was normal to get food poisoning so often.

It took a massive vertigo attack to finally break me down and force me to admit that I needed help. What happened next was undeniable.

My girlfriend Megan and I had just finished eating dinner. As a typical college student, my diet at the time largely consisted of nutritional garbage. On this particular night, the fast food du jour was a bacon cheeseburger with fries.

After we had finished eating, I stood up to throw away the trash, when suddenly a massive wave of vertigo hit me all at once and knocked me back onto the couch. The room started to spin. My tinnitus was louder than I would ever have thought was possible. Pressure filled my ear and it became very hard to hear. The room spun faster and faster. I could barely move as the nausea took over. I'm lucky that I was standing next to the couch and not on a staircase when it hit, and I'm lucky that Megan was there to help.

But Megan was powerless to make it stop. We didn't even know what was happening. All she could do was run her fingers through my hair and tell me, "We're going to get you help. It's all going to be okay." She had been urging me to see a doctor for weeks, but I had always refused. I was confident that whatever was going on would either disappear or get better over time. But as I sat shivering on the couch, panic coursing through my veins, I realized how mistaken I was. Something was very wrong with me. I promised Megan I would go to the doctor as soon as possible.

I was diagnosed with Meniere's disease shortly after this final incident. But my first doctor delivered the diagnosis like a death sentence, completely devoid of any empathy or compassion. He refused to answer any of my questions or consider alternatives. But I didn't know any better at the time. Why would I suspect he could be wrong about an illness I knew nothing about? It was a hard pill to swallow.

I truly believed my life was over, and as I continued to do my own research, the confusing, often conflicting information I found on the internet only made everything worse. It was one of the darkest hours of my entire life. I had no hope. Accepting an incurable illness with such severe symptoms and harsh limitations is devastatingly difficult.

But slowly, I pulled myself out of my funk and started taking action. I found an amazing specialist who confirmed the diagnosis with a series of tests and I resolved to do everything in my power to fight my way back to health.

I still have Meniere's disease, and until medical science comes up with a cure, I always will. But I did get my life back. If your tinnitus is caused by Meniere's disease, I want you to know that there is so much hope for you too. I encourage you to visit my Meniere's disease blog, MindOverMenieres.com to learn more, and to check out my first book, *Mind Over Meniere's: How I Conquered Meniere's Disease and Learned to Thrive.*

# My Tinnitus

It has now been more than five years since my Meniere's diagnosis, and I'm happy to say that I haven't had a vertigo attack in a very long time. Megan and I married, I started a business, and I found ways to live a life of passion and purpose.

But it's not all rosy all the time. I do still struggle with Meniere's disease. I may not have had an attack recently, but I do get dizzy from time to time. I still get the feeling of pressure in my ears, and I still have tinnitus. In fact, my tinnitus was the one symptom that never really improved. Meniere's disease made it considerably worse, and as my Meniere's got better, my tinnitus stayed the same.

For a long time, I just tried to ignore it. I blasted white noise and nature sounds when I went to sleep. I listened to music while I worked, and I avoided silence like the plague. But my tinnitus continued to bother me. Once again, it was making my life a living hell and becoming impossible to ignore.

My tinnitus is a loud, high-pitched tone with a frequency of around 3500 Hertz that never goes away. When my Meniere's symptoms flare up, however, I do hear other sounds. Over the years I've heard higher pitched tones, lower pitched tones, whooshing sounds, static, and more, but the high-pitched tone is always with me. It's loud enough to drive me crazy all on its own, and during flare-ups it would become unbearable. I tried every "cure" I could get my hands on: Lipo-flavinoids, bioflavonoids, vitamins, tinnitus supplements, and more. Nothing ever worked, and I suffered for a long time. It was the one thing I had no control over.

It wasn't until much later that I discovered something that actually helped. There is still no cure for tinnitus as I write this, but at the same time, my tinnitus no longer bothers me at all. A simple exercise changed everything. My focus improved, the anxiety my tinnitus was causing me disappeared, and I can now even fall asleep without white noise. At last, silence is no longer my enemy.

But before I get into the details, you need to understand what tinnitus is, what causes it, and how it can become such a problem.

# Chapter 2

# What Exactly Is Tinnitus?

"The strongest people I've met have not been given an easier life. They've learned to create strength and happiness from dark places."

- Kristen Butler, founder of Power of Positivity

First things first, let's start with the medical definition. According to the Mayo Clinic, "Tinnitus is the perception of noise or ringing in the ears…Tinnitus isn't a condition itself — it's a symptom of an underlying condition."

Unfortunately, there are quite a few underlying conditions that cause tinnitus. It's an extremely common medical phenomenon. Just to give you an idea, hearing loss (both age-related and noise-induced), injury (both to the ear, and to the head and neck), Temporomandibular Joint Disorder (TMJ), traumatic brain injury, infection, vestibular disorders like Meniere's disease, Migraine Associated Vertigo (MAV) and Superior Semicircular Canal Dehiscence Syndrome (SCDS), and circulatory system disorders are all known to cause tinnitus. Certain vitamins, supplements, and medications can cause tinnitus, too. In his book, *I Can Live with Tinnitus*, author Roger Bray explains, "Numerous prescription and non-prescription drugs list tinnitus as a side effect. Some of the most common are aspirin and quinine. Sedatives, anti-depressants, antibiotics, cancer medications and anti-inflammatories are also common causes. Higher doses of any of these medications can increase the chances of tinnitus and/or make it worse."

It's safe to say that there are a lot of roads that lead to tinnitus. But at the end of the day, how you got it is less important than how you choose to deal with it.

Finding a doctor, whether an audiologist, otolaryngologist (an ear, nose, and throat doctor), or a neurologist, who is knowledgeable about tinnitus and aware of the various treatment options, is a top priority. It's important to find a doctor with an uplifting personality, one who leaves you with a sense of hope and optimism. In my experience, this makes all the difference.

It's also important to rule out any potentially treatable medical conditions that could be causing your tinnitus. For example, if it's caused by hearing loss, hearing aids can sometimes offer dramatic improvements. An audiologist can quickly check your hearing with a simple test called an audiogram, and fit hearing aids if necessary.

You can find a great local doctor by searching on Healthgrades.com. In the last few years, doctor rating websites have become somewhat commonplace, but Healthgrades is my personal favorite. It lists the conditions that each doctor treats, any malpractice suits or awards the doctor may have, and offers a five-star rating system based on anonymous patient feedback and surveys.

We now have a general description of tinnitus, and the underlying conditions that are known to cause it. It's a good starting point, but it doesn't really offer us anything useful. And the majority of tinnitus sufferers never learn anything beyond this.

To understand what tinnitus actually is, and how it can become so problematic, we have to take a closer look at the physical structure of the ear, and examine how we process sound in the first place.

## This Is Your Brain on Sound

The hearing process begins when sound waves enter the ear canal and hit the eardrum, which transmits the sound waves as vibrations to the middle ear. Next, in the middle ear, three tiny bones - the malleus (hammer), the incus (anvil), and the stapes (stirrup) - convert the vibrations into physical waves that ripple through the fluid-filled cochlea in the inner ear.

The cochlea is a small snail-shaped organ that translates the waves into electrical signals the brain can understand. These signals are then sent as nerve impulses to the auditory cortex, the region of the brain that processes sound. Our brain is able to identify a sound by matching the electrical patterns with familiar patterns from memory. In the case of tinnitus, this is where the problems arise.

Whenever we hear a sound for the first time, we don't just label it, we also assign meaning, and react accordingly. The meaning we assign, and the way we react, depends entirely on how it makes us feel, and whether we believe that the sound implies something positive or negative. Later on, if we hear the sound again, we don't just remember what the sound was, but also what it means, and how it made us feel.

This process has actually played an important role in our survival as a species. We use sound to monitor our environment for threats. For example, when our prehistoric ancestors heard the growl of a saber-toothed tiger in the middle of the night, a sound they would have known well, the meaning was always clear: danger. And when danger strikes, we are wired to react in a specific way. As a result, the growl of a tiger would automatically trigger the "fight or flight" response, giving our ancestors a chance to face the threat, or get away safely.

This panicked, anxiety-provoking stress response doesn't feel very good while it's happening, but it does serve a purpose: It primes the body to react to danger. For a brief period of time, we can run faster, hit harder, and see more clearly. Our senses become heightened, our hearing more acute.

But at the same time, it's not all about identifying threats either. Sounds can also carry a deeply positive association. It's why we feel happy when we listen to music we love, and why we find the sounds of nature so relaxing. It's also why a baby is soothed by the sound of its mother's voice.

So now we have two pieces of the puzzle: memory and meaning. When a sound is important enough or carries enough of an emotional impact, we assign meaning to it and react accordingly. The problem is, if our reaction to a sound is consistent, over time it becomes an automatic response that activates both the limbic system, triggering an emotional response, and the autonomic nervous system, causing a physical response in the body. Very quickly a sound can become so closely intertwined with a specific response that, when we hear it, we react automatically without thinking at all.

It's why a mother will be jolted awake by the sound of her crying baby, even though she may have slept through a noisy storm. It's why the growl of a tiger instantly triggers the fight or flight response, and why we will suddenly jump to attention at the sound of our name heard softly across a crowded room.

It's also why tinnitus can become such a problem: When it is perceived as an annoyance or a threat, our body reacts automatically as if we were in danger, triggering a stress response.

But the reality is that tinnitus is no more threatening or dangerous than the sound of a ceiling fan.

So what exactly is tinnitus?

## A Reason for Hope

According to the Neurophysiological Model of Tinnitus, developed by Dr. Jonathan Hazel and Dr. Pawel Jastreboff in the early 1990s, the answer starts with a closer look at the cochlea. Within the cochlea sound waves are translated into electrical nerve impulses via 17,000 tiny hair-shaped sensory organs, called hair cells. A lot is going on inside the cochlea, and it happens to be a very noisy environment. In fact, the mechanical and electrical activity within the cochlea, combined with the constant movement of the hair cells, produces a measurable noise. These sounds are known as otoacoustic emissions, and can be recorded with sensitive microphones.

This is important to understand, because it means that even people who don't have tinnitus can hear the sounds of tinnitus under the right conditions. And we've known this for over 60 years.

In 1953, two scientists named Heller and Bergman conducted a clever experiment that has since been replicated several times. They recruited 80 university students with no history of tinnitus, and led them to believe they were having their hearing tested. Inside a sound absorbing (anechoic) booth, the students were instructed to press a button whenever they heard any sounds played through their headphones.

But it was a trick. For five straight minutes, no sounds were played at all, and yet incredibly, 93% of the students pressed the button. When questioned afterward, the students reported hearing a wide range of sounds, including buzzing, pulsing, and whistling noises. The **exact** sounds reported by most tinnitus sufferers.

Heller and Bergman demonstrated that just about everyone is capable of hearing the background electrical and mechanical noise present in the cochlea, in the inner ear, and in the nerve cells throughout our hearing pathways.

Tinnitus is therefore not something dangerous, or threatening, or a sign of internal damage. It's the result of your brain turning up the volume of natural sounds present within the body, sounds that everyone can hear under the right conditions. Typically, this happens as your brain attempts to compensate for changes in your sound environment such as silence, hearing loss, or exposure to sudden noise. It's an overcompensation, but a natural process nonetheless.

As a side note, hyperacusis, or extreme sensitivity to sound, happens when your brain turns up the volume of certain external sounds in your environment, as opposed to the internal sounds of tinnitus. But it's a closely related phenomenon. 40% of tinnitus sufferers also report varying degrees of hyperacusis. The techniques and strategies I will teach you in part two of the book may help to improve this form of sensitivity as well.

Unfortunately, we still don't know why this overcompensation occurs, and we only have a rough idea of where tinnitus originates in the brain. Some researchers, like David Ryugo, a professor of neuroscience at the Garvan Institute in Sydney, Australia, theorize that when the brain experiences a reduction or change in auditory stimulation, it will find ways to fill the empty space. In an interview with journalist Jill Margo for the Australian Financial Review, Ryugo explains, "When the brain is no longer receiving good stimulation, it alters its expectations and rewires itself. Some of the space it previously dedicated to hearing begins being used for other functions... The brain doesn't like a vacuum, and just as amputees suffer phantom limb pain, so hearing loss can give rise to phantom sounds as tinnitus." But again, we don't really know why this happens or what underlying mechanisms are involved. There are still a large number of unanswered questions, and much more research is needed.

But the key takeaway here is that the sounds of tinnitus are harmless, no matter how loud they may seem, or how intrusive they are.

The only difference between someone who is tormented by the sound of their tinnitus, and someone who isn't bothered at all, is that the sufferer's brain perceives the sound as a threat, an annoyance, or as something dangerous, and develops a negative conditioned response of panic, anxiety, or stress.

The good news for the people who are tortured by their tinnitus is that the negative reaction can be reprogrammed, and replaced with a positive one.

Chapter 3

# Habituation Is the Answer

"The truth that many people never understand, until it is too late, is that the more you try to avoid suffering, the more you suffer, because smaller and more insignificant things begin to torture you, in proportion to your fear."

- Thomas Merton, writer and Trappist Monk

The human brain is very good at eliminating distracting and meaningless background noise from our conscious awareness. It's why we're able to focus and work in noisy environments, like a busy sales office or a coffee shop. It's also how we're able to carry on conversations in loud restaurants. This mental process is known as habituation and in a very real sense, the brain is able to turn down the volume of sounds that aren't important so we can focus on the ones that are. We do this automatically, all the time.

Habituation is also the key to living with tinnitus, but there's a big problem. It's simply not possible to habituate to a sound that implies a threat, an annoyance, or if it carries a negative association of any kind. After all, you would never want to be able to tune out the sound of a fire alarm in the middle of the night, or any other noises that imply danger, for that matter.

It is possible to habituate to the sound of your tinnitus, the people who live comfortably with their tinnitus all have, but you have to first defuse your negative response to the sound. Otherwise, you will continue to react automatically, both physically and emotionally, as if you were in danger, preventing habituation from ever happening naturally.

So now the question is, how did we develop such a negative response to the sound of our tinnitus? And why would we perceive it as a threat if it isn't one?

The negative conditioning usually starts with fear. The sudden onset of a disturbing noise that no one else can hear can be terrifying, especially when you don't know what's going on. I was scared out of my mind the first time Meniere's disease cranked up the volume. A lot of people panic and believe that something is terribly wrong with them. Most people can tolerate a temporary problem, but when the sound doesn't go away, the stress and the fear continue to build. The sound of silence is also something we treasure, and we grieve when it's taken away.

If you're anything like me, you may have taken to the internet to search for answers, only to find terrible words like "incurable" and "forever" being tossed around with reckless abandon. The panic intensifies as the perceived threat becomes more real and more permanent, causing the conditioned response to grow stronger. Depression will often settle in and sleep becomes difficult.

Most people's first instinct is to try to ignore it, either by force of will or by distracting themselves with TV, music, or ambient noise. It certainly was for me. If you still have your hearing, background noise can help to block it out. But it doesn't address the underlying problem, and can make everything worse in the long run. Never in my life have I witnessed someone solve a problem by ignoring it, yet for some reason, that's what so many of us try to do. Emotional, physical, and psychological problems all get worse when we ignore them. So why do we think it will be any different when it comes to tinnitus? When people try to ignore the sound of their tinnitus, they usually only succeed in feeling more frustrated, anxious, and afraid. And over time, it can end up doing more harm than good.

The problem is that our brains can't tell the difference between a perceived threat, like tinnitus, and real danger. As a result, we end up in a perpetual low-level state of fight or flight, which if you recall, heightens our senses. Our hearing gets sharper, which causes the tinnitus to seem louder. And the harder we try to ignore it, the harder our brains fight to redirect our attention to the source of the perceived threat by turning up the volume even more. Put simply, the more we try to ignore it, the worse it gets.

We also start to associate the sound of our tinnitus with our feelings of frustration, strengthening the negative conditioning even further. For so many of us, the sound becomes a constant source of stress and emotional turmoil. We try to ignore it, but can't, continuously fueling our frustration in a never-ending vicious cycle.

And doctors don't always help either. Too many of us have been told that we simply have to live with it, and that is not constructive advice. Many practicing doctors just don't have the time to stay up to date on the latest research and treatment protocols, while others are so desperately lacking in empathy and compassion that the patient is left feeling hopeless.

When faced with such adversity, it's hard to believe that anyone can learn to live with their tinnitus. The odds are definitely not in our favor. But this is the reality of our situation and one that untold millions of people face on a daily basis.

I know I've painted a dark picture, but hopefully by now you can understand that there is hope, regardless of what your tinnitus sounds like. Every single one of us has the capacity to habituate to the sound of our tinnitus. And when we do, it may not go away, but it will stop bothering us.

# Neuroplasticity and Rewiring the Brain

The human brain is one of the most powerful information processing machines in the universe, but we're born without an instruction manual. It makes you wonder how fewer problems we might have if the Western world became more interested in learning to manage the mind.

In fact, the brain is capable of incredible feats of healing. Under the right circumstances, the brain can forge new neural pathways, literally rewiring itself to various beneficial ends. This is known as neuroplasticity, or brain plasticity, and refers to the field of research that has shown that the brain is not fixed, but remains changeable throughout our entire life. In other words, there is a biological basis for habituation. If our brains were fixed, we would be unable to reprogram our response to the sound of our tinnitus.

So to summarize – we know that tinnitus becomes a problem when we develop an automatic negative conditioned response to the sound, and that habituation is the answer, but it is only possible when there is no negative association.

The next step is to take the specific actions that cause this shift in association to happen. The plan is simple. First, I will teach you techniques to not only eliminate your negative response but replace it with one that is emotionally positive, one that will enable habituation to happen naturally. I will also give you specific tools, techniques, and strategies to accelerate the natural habituation process. By cherry picking the best components of other tinnitus treatment strategies and therapies, and combining them in a new and powerful way, I will show you how I was able to drastically speed up the time it took me to habituate.

In my experience, these techniques have the potential to work very quickly, but I want to be clear. This is not a miracle cure. It will take hard work, discipline, and courage, but if you stick with it, you can start to improve. I will walk you through the process step by step, and give you everything you need to finally get the relief you so desperately deserve. When you habituate, your tinnitus may not go away, but it will stop bothering you, and you will stop reacting to it. As you start this journey, I want you to know that you are not alone and that there is so much hope.

Let's begin!

# Part 2:
# Rapid Habituation

# Chapter 4

# The Backstory

"You either get bitter or you get better. It's that simple. You either take what has been dealt to you and allow it to make you a better person, or you allow it to tear you down. The choice does not belong to fate, it belongs to you."

- Josh Shipp, author and youth speaker

When I was first diagnosed with Meniere's disease, my doctor told me that I needed to lower my stress levels. He explained that stress would make all my symptoms, including tinnitus, a lot worse, and that if I wanted to improve, I needed to find a better way to calm down. But I had lived with terrible anxiety for a long time, and being diagnosed with a rare and incurable illness that can make you go deaf is no cake walk. I was swallowed whole by an anxious abyss.

For most of my adult life, I had relied on various medications to manage my anxiety. It helped the physical symptoms and prevented panic attacks, but it never addressed the underlying issues that were causing the problem in the first place. Over the years, I did try to manage my anxiety in other ways, but only somewhat successfully. Therapy, for example, had helped me up to a point, but never enough to make me feel that I was ready to stop taking anxiety medications. For a long time, I just lived with it and continued taking the medications to get me through the day. I knew it wasn't sustainable, but at the time I didn't feel I had a choice.

What ended up working for me was learning how to meditate, though I must admit it took a long time for me to actually try it. I was very skeptical initially, and when I finally gave it a shot, I almost quit right away. I found it difficult and frustrating, and I didn't really know what I was doing. I also wasn't the only one struggling with all these issues. Most people who decide to try meditation seem to go through something similar. In his New York Times bestselling book, *10% Happier,* author and ABC News anchorman Dan Harris summed up my skepticism perfectly, "Meditation suffers from a towering PR problem, largely because its most prominent proponents talk as if they have a perpetual pan flute accompaniment. If you can get past the cultural baggage, though, what you'll find is that meditation is simply exercise for your brain." Looking back, I'm somewhat surprised that I stuck with it, but also very grateful that I did.

Perhaps at this point it might be helpful to provide

a clear definition of meditation. Simply put,
practice of quieting the mind. Typically, this ⸺ʌ⸗ʋıves
focusing your attention onto a single point of awareness,
like your breathing, or a mantra, which is a mentally
repeated word or phrase.

Many people are under the impression that their
thoughts and mental chatter are outside their control.
After all, who would willingly choose to face that
constant whirlwind of reminders, insight, negative self-
talk, and random bits of narrative. Most people don't
realize that it's even possible to quiet their mind and
silence their inner voice. But that's exactly what
meditation has to offer and so much more.

In the short term, meditation triggers a relaxation
response that calms the nervous system and, as a result,
the body and mind. It also causes an immediate
reduction in stress. But it's the long-term effects that are
the most desirable. Overall stress levels start to go down
while the ability to cope with stress becomes stronger.
Focus and concentration improve dramatically. When
stress does occur, you are able to center and calm
yourself much more quickly. You begin to react less and
respond more. The ability to quiet the mind also allows
you to fall asleep faster and more easily.

I struggled for a while with meditation but I didn't
give up, and at some point I realized that I needed a

more structured approach. Whatever I was doing wasn't working. I started reading about the different styles of meditation, trying each one to see how it fit. I tried guided meditations, mantra meditation, mindfulness, and more. Sometimes, I would just focus my attention and awareness on my breathing, or a part of my body, like my stomach. Other times I would try to simply observe my thoughts as they popped into my head. I also learned how to use self-hypnosis techniques to go into the deep state of relaxation known as the trance state. Basically, it's an altered state of consciousness where your body falls asleep, but your mind remains awake and aware. It's wild; every muscle in your body becomes completely relaxed, and at times you can even feel your eyes fluttering in Rapid Eye Movement (REM). Even my fitness tracking watch would record me as being in REM sleep, though I was consciously aware the entire time.

I gradually started to develop my own style and find a rhythm with meditation. I was also starting to really enjoy it, and began to look forward to it every day. More importantly, though, I was seeing results. My anxiety was definitely showing signs of improvement. It all seemed so promising. Throughout the day, I felt more relaxed, more of the time, and it seemed as though the habit was finally starting to stick. I practiced every day for months and months. I was even able to wean off my anxiety medications. But after a year or so of progress, I started to slip up. As my workload and responsibilities increased, my meditation practice suffered, until eventually I stopped meditating altogether.

For a while, things remained stable. But a few months later, I was diagnosed with Meniere's disease, and the anxiety returned with a vengeance. Fortunately, I felt prepared this time around and knew how to handle it. I started meditating right away, and I guess it was the right decision because I did improve, both emotionally and psychologically.

In hindsight, I don't think I would ever have adjusted to Meniere's disease as well as I was able to were it not for meditation. I also found that it helped me manage the stress that my tinnitus was causing me once my other Meniere's symptoms started to improve. The only problem was that my tinnitus made it extremely difficult to focus. No matter how hard I tried to ignore it, it kept messing with my meditation. I felt frustrated and lost, and I wasn't sure what to do about it. I knew that meditation was helping me, but it was getting harder to manage.

## The Breakthrough

I continued to meditate daily, but my tinnitus was getting worse. It got so bad, in fact, that I started to dread meditation and almost stopped entirely. I scoured the internet for answers, desperately looking for something I could use, something that would help me ignore the ringing so that I could focus. Nothing seemed to work.

At some point though, while lying in bed struggling to meditate, I suddenly had an idea. Everyone always tries to ignore their tinnitus, but it never works. What would happen, I wondered, if I tried the opposite? It occurred to me that I was bothered by my tinnitus the most when I actively tried to ignore it, but couldn't. So instead of trying to block it out, what if I consciously and intentionally focused on the sound? If meditation involved focusing my attention onto a single point of awareness, like my breathing, why couldn't I focus on the ringing instead? And by extension, if I used the sound of my tinnitus for meditation, and focused on it by choice, would it possibly start to bother me less throughout the day? I had no idea, and to be honest, I was somewhat scared to find out. Focusing on the sound that was driving me crazy seemed crazy, but I also had the feeling that I might have stumbled onto something interesting, something new. After a few minutes, my curiosity got the best of me, and I gave it a shot. It was the one thing my brain and my tinnitus never expected me to do, and it changed everything.

The first surprise was that it was actually quite

difficult to put into practice, but not for the reasons I was expecting. As soon as I tried to focus on the sound, my mind would start to wander. Truth be told, this is what happens with all forms of meditation. The goal of meditation is not to keep your mind empty and focused at all times, but to gently bring your focus back when you catch your mind drifting. Yet when my mind wandered during the tinnitus focused meditation, it wandered away from the sound. Much to my delight, for those brief moments of distraction, my tinnitus didn't bother me at all. It was the first in a series of major breakthroughs, and I finished meditating with a huge grin on my face. After just one session, I was shocked to find that the ringing seemed much quieter for a while. No, that wasn't it, the ringing was still there. It just wasn't bothering me as much, so it didn't seem as loud.

I couldn't explain why it was happening, but my tinnitus seemed to lose some of its power over me, and as I continued to practice, it continued to improve. It all seemed so counterintuitive. Eventually, I came to understand what was happening and why, but at the time all that mattered was that it was working.

It also changed the way I thought about tinnitus, and I suddenly found myself flooded with new insights, ideas and theories. I experimented constantly, and over time, I discovered ways to make my tinnitus focused meditation even more effective. Slowly but surely, this simple technique that I had stumbled upon by accident evolved into a powerful framework for treating my tinnitus.

## Tinnitus Doesn't Have to Be a Bad Thing

At the end of the day, habituating to the sound of your tinnitus is a matter of rewiring your emotional response. Remember, the goal is to not only eliminate your negative response to the sound but to replace it with a new, emotionally positive reaction. And while some people do habituate naturally over time, for everyone else the best strategy is to turn the sound of their tinnitus into something useful, something positive. Tinnitus focused meditation accomplishes all of this and more.

If you're feeling skeptical or having a hard time wrapping your mind around this, I completely understand. When my tinnitus was at its worst, if you had told me that one day I wouldn't mind having tinnitus, I would have thought you were insane. How could something that caused me so much pain and so much anxiety ever be anything but negative?

The bottom line is that meditation makes it possible. Because meditation is such a powerfully relaxing practice with the ability to calm the nervous system, and because anything can be used as the focal point of meditation, even something as problematic as tinnitus can be used to our advantage.

Again, in his book *10% Happier*, Dan Harris offers an explanation of how this is possible as he gives advice on dealing with boredom, a common problem experienced during meditation, "The advice here is similar to how you should handle pain and fatigue: Investigate. What does boredom feel like? How does it manifest in your body? Whatever comes up in your mind can be co-opted and turned into the object of meditation. It's like in judo, where you use the force of your enemy against him."

But tinnitus meditation can also enable the habituation process to occur. As you practice, your brain starts to associate the deep relaxation of meditation with the sound of your tinnitus, completely overwriting your negative conditioned response. Once that happens, there is nothing to prevent you from habituating naturally. And at some point, you will suddenly realize that hours, or even days, have passed where you didn't think about your tinnitus at all.

Tinnitus meditation also offers you a way to stop ignoring the sound of your tinnitus and finally face it head on. By choosing to focus on the sound on your own terms, and on your schedule, you will start to focus on it less the rest of the time.

## Using What Works

Around this time, I also took a closer look at what else was being done to treat tinnitus around the world. I knew that I wasn't the only person to habituate. I wanted to learn more about what other people were doing. Surprisingly, I found that there weren't a whole lot of options available to most tinnitus sufferers. In some cases, doctors didn't seem to offer any solutions at all. But for the ones that did, Tinnitus Retraining Therapy (TRT) was one of the most common approaches.

The goal of TRT, like my strategy, is to enable the person to habituate to the sound of their tinnitus. And it's not just a way to mask the symptoms; it actually addresses the underlying issues that prevent habituation from happening naturally. The problem is that it takes anywhere from 6 to 24 months to see results. That's a long time, and it requires a lot of hard work and commitment to make it to the finish line. To facilitate habituation, TRT takes a three-pronged approach. First, the patient is educated by their doctor on the ins and outs of tinnitus. After education, the patient is fitted with expensive sound masking devices that look like hearing aids but play white noise directly into the ear at a volume that partially masks the sound of their tinnitus. The idea here is that if you can reduce the perceived volume of tinnitus to a more tolerable level, it won't bother the patient as much, and will allow habituation to occur over time. Lastly, TRT also involves the use of Cognitive Behavioral Therapy (CBT) to help the patient replace the emotionally negative response with one that is emotionally neutral.

TRT has unquestionably helped a lot of people, but it's not without its limitations. For starters, it won't work if you have hearing loss. Obviously, if you can't hear the masking sound, you won't be able to reduce the perceived volume. This setback applies to all sound-masking-based approaches to treating tinnitus. It also takes a long time to see results, though the time investment isn't a limiting factor or barrier to entry. It just makes it harder to succeed, because it requires so much of you for such a long period of time. The real problem is that it's expensive, and the monetary investment is a barrier to entry for a huge portion of the population. The doctor visits, the expensive equipment, and the months and years of therapy all cost money, and that money adds up quickly.

The good news is that there are several aspects of TRT that work quite well and can be freely used to your advantage. As I experimented with tinnitus meditation, I discovered that some of the principals of TRT, like the concept of partial masking, can make the practice much easier, and more accessible to sufferers with severe cases of tinnitus. My goal was to create a system that was not only more powerful but also financially accessible to the masses.

As I continued my research, I was able to pull the best ideas from a wide range of other disciplines and treatment strategies. The end result is a comprehensive system that can be adapted to work for everyone, regardless of the severity of their tinnitus, or whether or not they have hearing loss.

With Tinnitus Retraining Therapy, habituation is eventually able to occur because you learn to experience your tinnitus as something harmless. But it takes a long time. With tinnitus meditation, you're able to transform the sound of your tinnitus into something useful right from the start, which can speed up the process of habituation exponentially.

By the end of this chapter, you will have a clear path forward. And if you stick with it, you can habituate to the sound of your tinnitus. You're already closer than you could possibly imagine. It's time for your tinnitus to stop bothering you.

# Chapter 5

# The Tinnitus Meditation Protocol

"You can't calm the storm, so stop trying. What you can do is calm yourself. The storm will pass."

- Timber Hawkeye, author

B efore we begin, I want to let you know that while the basic tinnitus meditation techniques are accessible to everyone, I'm also going to give you tools and teach you a variety of other techniques that may or may not be helpful, depending on your individual circumstances. These additional techniques are designed to either make tinnitus meditation easier, more effective, or to speed up the habituation process, and they are helpful when you're first starting out. But if you have significant hearing loss, for example, you won't be able to take advantage of any audio based tools.

Everyone experiences tinnitus differently. Some people have hearing loss, others have hyperacusis, and no two individuals hear exactly the same sound. Once you have learned all the different techniques, you will have a much better idea of what will work best for your individual needs.

I recommend that you first finish reading the rest of the book before attempting any of the techniques. It will give you a better grasp of the overall strategy. And even if you find that some of the techniques or tools don't apply to you, it's still an important step. It will give you a better understanding of what you are up against, and at the end of the book, I will provide you with a step by step action plan.

I also want to address a concern that some of you may still have: Focusing on the sound of your tinnitus inherently feels like a bad idea. There's a good reason you might feel this way. As we learned earlier, all the problematic aspects of your tinnitus - the anxiety, fear, stress, insomnia, distress, and everything else in between - have become a conditioned and automatic response to the sound. Just thinking about tinnitus can be enough to trigger these emotions, and I know that for some of you, reading this much about tinnitus may have been difficult.

All I ask is that you keep an open mind.

# First Contact Journaling Exercise

The first step in your treatment is a simple journaling exercise designed to help you explore the sound of your tinnitus. It will give you both the chance to experience it from a new perspective and a closer look at what's actually going on. All you need is a blank sheet of paper, something to write with, and a quiet space.

After reading about the technique, if you don't think you are ready to handle it just yet, I will provide you with a set of tools in the next chapter that will make this much easier. The same goes for the tinnitus meditation technique.

## Journaling Exercise:

I want you to close your eyes and imagine that you are hearing the sound of your tinnitus for the very first time. On a sheet of paper, describe it in as much detail as you possibly can. Approach this from the mindset of a curious observer, or a scientist describing an exciting new discovery to his colleagues. It can also be helpful to imagine that you are writing a letter to your loved ones to describe the sound of your tinnitus, so that they will better understand what you're going through.

On the sheet of paper, answer as many of the following questions as possible:

1. What does your tinnitus sound like?
   a. Does it sound like something familiar, or anything else that you can think of?
   b. Is it a single tone, or multiple tones?
   c. Does it sound like chirping or buzzing? Maybe it's more of a whooshing sound?
   d. Can you identify more than one noise?
   e. As you listen, do the sounds change at all or do they remain constant?
2. Where does it feel like the sound is coming from?
   a. Is it in your ears, or in your head?
   b. Or does it sound like it's coming from somewhere else entirely, as if you were near a radio?
   c. And how loud does it seem to be?
   d. Does the volume change at all or is it steady?

Feel free to use colorful language and write down as much as you can. Once you have a solid description, I want you to close your eyes again and look inward.

3. How does it make you feel, both mentally and physically?
   a. Do you feel any anxiety, stress, pain, or discomfort?

    b. Take a minute to mentally focus on each part of your body. Do you feel anything specific in any part of your body? Maybe you feel it as tension in your stomach or your chest? Maybe you feel it as lightheadedness or dizziness? Whatever you feel, maintain the mindset of a curious observer, and write down all of your thoughts.

4. Take a moment to explore your emotions in relation to tinnitus.

    a. Do you feel sad or angry, fearful or worried?

    b. Do you feel anything that could be considered a positive emotion? Maybe you feel a sense of apathy or ambivalence?

    c. Whatever you feel, describe the emotions but also try to look deeper to see what's behind them. Try to explain why you think you feel that way.

When you finish, I want you to read it back to yourself. It may not seem like very much, but you have just taken a huge first step. You have faced your tinnitus in a way that you probably never have before, and that's no small feat. You should be proud of this accomplishment, and I want you to know that you are well on your way toward habituation.

As a side note, it can be helpful to share what you've written with your loved ones. They probably don't have a very good idea of what you are going through, and sharing what you've written will help them understand. Plus, bringing your family and friends into the fold as you embark on this journey will help you on several levels. When you struggle, they can help keep you on the path, and give you the encouragement you need to keep going. They can also help to keep you accountable, to make sure that you stick to your practice schedule and routines.

Now that you have faced your tinnitus head on, you are ready to learn the tinnitus meditation technique.

# The Tinnitus Meditation Technique

The overall strategy here will involve more than the technique that I'm about to teach you, but everything else is secondary. If the tinnitus meditation technique is all you ever practice, you can still get the results you're looking for. It's the foundation on which everything else is built.

You also don't need to have any prior experience with meditation for it to work. Having experience with meditation will speed up the learning curve, but it's not a requirement. And while it's easy to learn, like most types of meditation, it requires practice. I'll walk you through the technique step by step.

To practice tinnitus meditation, you will not need to sit cross-legged on a yoga mat with a flower in your hair, chanting "om". What's important is that you're comfortable. Tinnitus meditation can be done sitting in a chair, on the floor, on the couch, or lying down. Your first order of business is just to get comfortable and make sure that there won't be any distractions. You're also going to need a timer. If your phone has one built in, that's perfect; just make sure to set it on airplane mode so you won't be interrupted. Otherwise, you can always just set an alarm to go off after a period of time.

I also want to stress that the goal here is not to maintain perfect focus or to keep your mind clear the entire time. When your mind starts to wander, and it will, it doesn't mean you're doing it wrong. This happens to everyone, especially new meditators, and with all types of meditation. Catching yourself when your mind wanders, and gently bringing your focus back to the sound, **is the exercise**. In her book, *Lovingkindness: The Revolutionary Art of Happiness*, author and meditation expert Sharon Salzberg explains, "Beginning again and again is the actual practice, not a problem to overcome so that one day we can come to the 'real' meditation." Also, it's important to face any unwanted thoughts or strange sensations you may experience without judgement. Never be hard on yourself. When your mind wanders, simply let the thought go and gently refocus your awareness. With practice, you will find that you can maintain your focus for longer and longer periods of time.

If you've never meditated before, it's best to start with a small obtainable goal and set your timer for five to ten minutes. If you are an experienced meditator, you can try this for as long as you'd like; just decide beforehand and set a timer.

The technique will start with a simple progressive muscle relaxation routine. When your body is completely relaxed, your mind will follow. It will help to calm you and lower your anxiety before you begin to focus on the sound of your tinnitus.

## Tinnitus Meditation:

Close your eyes and take five deep breaths into your diaphragm (lower abdomen). Feel your stomach expand as you inhale, and with each exhale, feel your entire body become more and more relaxed, letting all of your muscles go completely limp like a ragdoll.

Next, focus on relaxing individual muscle groups, one at a time, relaxing each as much as possible before moving on. Let all of the tension go as you work your way through your body.

Start by focusing on your feet and your toes. Allow the muscles to go completely limp. Now focus on your legs and your butt, releasing all the tension. Continue on to your stomach and your lower back, then your chest and upper back, your shoulders and your arms, your hands and your fingers, your neck and your throat, and finally, your head and your face.

Once you've worked your way through your body, and your muscles are completely relaxed, take another five deep breaths into your diaphragm.

Once your body is completely relaxed, it's time to focus your attention on the sound of your tinnitus. Try to maintain a mindset of curiosity, as if you were observing something interesting for the first time. Continue to breathe naturally and keep your mind focused on the sound. When your mind starts to wander, and you notice it happening, gently bring your focus back to the sound. Continue until the timer goes off.

As you continue to practice this technique, you will find yourself becoming more and more relaxed during the meditation. Not only can this speed up your process of habituation, but you're also getting all of the benefits of regular meditation, killing two birds with one stone.

In addition to the basic technique, I have two simple variations for you to explore. The first of which adds an element of visualization and imagination, the purpose of which is to show you that your perception of the sound of your tinnitus isn't as rigid as you might have believed. Give it a try, and if it doesn't work for you the first time around, don't give up! It's still serving a purpose. It will help you maintain your mindset of curiosity and will enable you to face your tinnitus at an even deeper level with less anxiety.

## Variation #1 – Visualization:

Start with the basic tinnitus meditation technique. Get comfortable, do the progressive muscle relaxation exercise, and begin to focus on the sound of your tinnitus.

As you focus on the sound, I want you to imagine that there is a large volume knob floating in front of you that can control the volume of your tinnitus. Imagine yourself playing with the volume knob, turning it up and down. You may be as surprised as I was to find that you can temporarily adjust the volume of the sound.

Next, I want you to imagine that there is a large on/off switch floating to the left of the volume knob. I like to imagine it as a giant circuit breaker switch with a big handle, similar to something a mad scientist would flip to turn on a large evil machine. Once you have the picture in your mind, imagine yourself flipping the switch on and off. Sometimes I like to imagine of a series of large switches that I shut down, one by one. Either way, I'm always surprised to find it produces a change in the sound of my tinnitus.

Now I want you to imagine a second knob, right next to the volume knob, that controls the tone of the sound. Visualize yourself turning this knob as well. My baseline tinnitus is a single high-frequency tone, but I'm able to temporarily lower and raise the pitch with this technique. You may find that you can do the same.

Spend a few minutes mentally turning the knobs and flipping switches. Pay close attention to any changes you hear in the sound of your tinnitus.

Finally, imagine that the sound of your tinnitus is actually coming from a speaker that is somewhere else in the room. Alternatively, you can imagine that another person is in the room with you, making the noise with their mouth. The source of the sound doesn't matter, as long as you imagine it as coming from somewhere else in the room. Once you have a clear sense of this in your mind, imagine the source of the sound exploding, or disappearing in a puff of smoke.

Continue to explore all these mental images until the timer goes off.

The second variation of the tinnitus meditation technique is designed to help you improve your control, while focusing your awareness. Your control will improve regardless, but this simple technique can speed up the process quite a bit.

## Variation #2 – Awareness Control:

Again, start with the basic tinnitus meditation technique. Get comfortable, do the progressive muscle relaxation exercise, and begin focusing on the sound.

Once you have a good rhythm going, expand your awareness to include everything else around you. This is known as mindfulness meditation. The idea is to stay focused on the object of your meditation, which in this case is the sound of your tinnitus, while simultaneously maintaining an awareness of everything else that is going on around you and within you.

Notice any sounds, or smells. Notice how you feel physically and emotionally. Are you feeling boredom, or pain, or discomfort? Explore it. For several minutes expand your awareness to include everything else. When you notice something, simply examine it, release it from your mind, and then refocus on the sound of your tinnitus.

The next step is to practice switching your focus from one point of awareness to another. For example, once you've expanded your awareness, you may have noticed the sound of your air conditioner quietly humming away in the background. For several breaths, focus on this new sound, making it the object of your meditation. Once you've done that, switch your focus back to the sound of your tinnitus for several breaths. Maybe you also noticed the scent of something from the kitchen, or a feeling of tension and anxiety in your stomach. For the next several breaths, you can make that the focal point of your meditation. Regardless of what you choose to focus on, as you change your point of awareness, only choose one thing at a time and try to tune everything else out.

You can hold your focus on each point of awareness for as long or as short as you like. Just make sure to go back to focusing on the sound of your tinnitus each time. Continue switching your focus back and forth until the timer goes off.

This will train you to focus your attention at will. By switching your focus from the sound of your tinnitus to a different point of awareness, and back again, your brain can learn to tune out the sound of your tinnitus when you aren't focusing on it.

Both variations are useful, and while you don't have to take advantage of them every time you practice tinnitus meditation, I've found that they add considerably to the experience, and help to keep it interesting. They can help to accelerate the habituation process too.

To make this as easy as possible for you, I have created guided tinnitus meditations for you to follow. They are part of a larger collection of audio tracks called the Tinnitus Relief Project designed to complement and enhance all the techniques found in the book. Visit Rewiringtinnitus.com/relief for more information.

Now that you have learned the basic tinnitus meditation techniques, we can build on that foundation. In the next chapter, I will draw on the latest research, treatment strategies, and related fields, to bring you a set of tools that can take your progress to the next level.

## Chapter 6

# Taking it Further

"It's not selfish to love yourself, take care of yourself, and make your happiness a priority."

— Mandy Hale, author

## Brainwave Entrainment

M ost people know that listening to a great song can change how they feel. But our emotional response to music is only one tiny aspect of its true potential. It goes much deeper. In fact, the technology exists to alter our mental state, and how we feel, in very targeted ways using nothing but sound. It's called Brainwave Entrainment, and it's becoming more powerful and more mainstream every day.

If you take this at face value for a moment, think of all the possibilities, especially for someone suffering from tinnitus. Imagine a song that could melt away your stress and anxiety, letting you face your tinnitus without fear. Or music that could put you in a deep meditative state automatically, even if you've never meditated before. All of this is possible, and more.

I should stress, however, that I will be focusing on audio based forms of Brainwave Entrainment technology, which will not work unless you have at least some of your hearing left in one of your ears. If this is a limiting factor for you, there are variations of this technology that use light, rather than sound, to alter consciousness. Visit Rewiringtinnitus.com/bookresources to learn more.

To understand how sound can possibly alter your consciousness in a significant way, I'll need to explain a few things. At any given moment in time, your brain is producing not one, but five different types of brainwaves: Delta, Theta, Alpha, Beta, and Gamma, each with their own unique frequency range. These electrical signals are how your brain cells communicate with each other, and one of the five is always more dominant than the rest. Which one it is depends on your mental state, how you feel, and whatever it is that you happen to be doing. Needless to say, this changes constantly. Right now, while you're reading, you are most likely in a Beta dominant brainwave state, which corresponds with wakefulness. Where specifically you fall within the Beta frequency range depends on how alert and focused you currently are.

The important thing to understand is that there is a specific, measurable, and somewhat predictable brainwave pattern directly associated with every action you could ever take, and with every single way you could possibly ever feel.

To put it simply, how you feel changes your brainwaves, yet surprisingly, the opposite is also true. You can change your mental state, and how you feel, by changing your brainwaves with an external stimulus. We are going to be doing this with sound.

Let's take a look, for example, at how this would work in the context of meditation. As it is with all mental states, during meditation our brainwaves change in a very predictable way.

Research, in which scientists use an EEG (electroencephalogram) to measure the brainwaves of Zen Buddhist monks in deep meditation, has shown this time and time again. For example, in one study published in the journal *Psychiatry and Clinical Neurosciences,* scientists found that while meditation changed the EEG results of participants with no Zen meditation training, the trained monks all experienced the same increase in Theta brainwave activity.

By engineering a Brainwave Entrainment audio

track to induce the same brainwave frequency patterns observed in the monks, you end up with what is essentially a guided meditation that communicates directly with your brain. As you listen to it, you will automatically experience the same deep level of meditation, and it only takes a few minutes to start working.

How it actually works is a little more complicated to understand. It starts with a strange phenomenon found in nature called the *Frequency Following Response* which describes a process by which similar patterns are able to synchronize with one another. For example, fireflies in large groups will synchronize their light flashes, while mosquitos flying together will synchronize the speed at which they flap their wings. Pendulum clocks hanging on the same wall, but set at different rates, will eventually synchronize their movements too. As will metronomes in close proximity.

But the Frequency Following Response also explains how certain types of sounds are able to influence brainwave patterns. When your brain is exposed to a steady rhythmic sound at a specific frequency, say seven beats per second (otherwise known as 7 Hertz), your brainwaves will begin to synchronize with the frequency of the beat. In this example, 7 Hertz, which happens to be a Theta brainwave frequency, temporarily becomes your dominant brainwave. And because 7 Hertz Theta brainwaves are closely correlated with feelings of stress relief, strong relaxation, and deep meditation, by simply listening to the sound of the beat, you will quickly find yourself feeling very relaxed.

So how can you use Brainwave Entrainment to help with your tinnitus? Some people listen to Brainwave Entrainment audio to mask the sound of their tinnitus and help them relax, but in my opinion, this doesn't actually solve anything and only offers temporary relief. Instead, you should use Brainwave Entrainment to ease the anxiety and negative emotions caused by your tinnitus, prior to tinnitus meditation, so that you can practice without fear or discomfort. You can also use Brainwave Entrainment to induce a deeper meditative state, allowing you to practice tinnitus meditation effectively, right from the very start. Both methods can help speed up the time it takes to habituate to the sound of your tinnitus, and enable you to start seeing results much more quickly.

There are several different types of Brainwave Entrainment audio, but I recommend Isochronic Tones. It's the newest and most powerful iteration of the technology, it works for people with partial hearing loss, and doesn't require the use of headphones. Other forms of audio-based Brainwave Entrainment, such as

Binaural Beats, won't work without headphones or if you have hearing loss.

I also want to offer a few words of caution. While the mind-altering effects of Brainwave Entrainment are never permanent, you should still be careful. Exposing yourself to audio embedded with the wrong brainwave frequencies can cause terrible headaches, as well as feelings of anxiety, fear, and panic. You're probably already experiencing these negative emotions from your tinnitus, and you definitely don't want to make matters worse. Accidentally inducing a panicked brainwave state while working to treat your tinnitus can bring your progress to a grinding halt. So while there may be many freely available Brainwave Entrainment audio tracks on YouTube, it's nearly impossible to know what you're getting. And that's unfortunate because an ineffective or poorly produced Brainwave Entrainment meditation track gives the technology a bad name. But when it's done right, the result is a rewarding and powerfully deep meditation experience. One that would ordinarily take time and rigorous daily practice to achieve.

For this reason, I have produced a set of powerful Brainwave Entrainment audio tracks specifically engineered for tinnitus as part of the Tinnitus Relief Project. There are tracks designed to alleviate your stress and anxiety before you practice tinnitus meditation, as well as others designed to be played while you meditate. Some of the tracks feature nature soundscapes, while others are mixed with relaxing meditation music, or calming white noise. The Tinnitus Relief Project is available at Rewiringtinnitus.com/relief.

If you are extremely agitated by the sound of your tinnitus, terrified by the prospect of tinnitus meditation, or even if you just simply want to relax, Brainwave Entrainment audio is the way to go. And it's easy to put into practice.

To reduce anxiety and relax prior to attempting the journaling exercise or tinnitus meditation, you just have to follow three easy steps.

First, select the track that you would like to listen to. They are all equally effective, but you may prefer to hear music or white noise rather than the sounds of nature. Simply listen to a minute or two of each track variation to see which version you like best. Once you have the track ready to go, the next step is to get comfortable. But be aware that these tracks are very sedating, and if you choose to lie down, you may fall asleep, defeating the purpose. In most cases, it's better to sit upright in a comfortable chair or on the couch. The last step is simply to press play, close your eyes, and listen. As long as you use headphones or a set of quality speakers, you will feel the effect within minutes. You can listen for as long as you like, and when you feel ready, just turn it off and complete the journaling exercise or begin to practice tinnitus meditation

Brainwave Entrainment is a safe, effective, and easy way to speed up your progress with tinnitus. Listening before you meditate can be extremely helpful, but if you want to use it during tinnitus meditation to induce a deeper meditative state, you have to take a slightly different approach, and further explanation is necessary.

## Partial Masking Exercises

One of the best aspects of Tinnitus Retraining Therapy is the concept of partial sound masking. If you recall, with TRT, the patient wears a hearing-aid-like device that plays white noise at a volume that partially masks the sound of their tinnitus. Blocking out some, but not all, of the sound of the patient's tinnitus, reduces their discomfort and allows them to habituate over time.

But you don't need expensive equipment or a long-term approach to take advantage of partial masking. There's a much easier way to put it into practice. One that can not only speed up the process of habituation, but can also enable sufferers with more severe cases of tinnitus to start taking action right away.

The technique is simple. All you have to do is use background noise - white noise, music, nature sounds, or any other ambient noise - to partially mask the sound of your tinnitus while you practice tinnitus meditation, or even while you complete your initial journaling exercise. The trick is to find the right balance of sound. You don't want to block out your perception of your tinnitus entirely; you just want to reduce it to a more comfortable level. To focus on the sound of your tinnitus during meditation, you will still need to be able to hear it. But if your tinnitus is overwhelming, you don't have to try to focus on it while it's blaring at full volume. Partial masking can help you get started with tinnitus meditation much more comfortably.

Regardless of what kind of ambient noise you use, I have two important guidelines. When you practice tinnitus meditation with partial masking, always make sure to:

1.  Use the lowest volume level of sound masking that you can tolerate.
2.  Only mask up to 70% of the sound of your tinnitus.

Partial sound masking is a great way to get started with tinnitus meditation and can drastically reduce your initial stress levels, but it's not a long-term solution.

Once you start to improve, you should slowly lower the volume of the masking sound. Remember, the goal is to get to the point where you have habituated to the sound of your tinnitus. To do that, you will eventually need to face your tinnitus at full volume. So, use partial masking, but begin to phase it out as soon as you feel comfortable doing so.

To put partial tinnitus masking to use, you have several good options. The first I've already covered, using ambient noise. But I also want to offer a slight variation of the technique that can be used to raise the difficulty level, once you get comfortable with the basic practice. It should be clear by now that challenging yourself at regular intervals is an important component of your overall strategy with tinnitus. It allows you to progress at a more rapid pace. So with this in mind, a simple twist on the partial masking strategy is to wear ear plugs.

Everyone with tinnitus knows that the noise is much louder in a quiet environment. Most of us tend to avoid silence like the plague. But wearing earplugs, while also playing ambient noise in the background to partially mask the sound of your tinnitus, works quite well. The earplugs will make your tinnitus louder while the ambient noise offers your brain something else to focus on, reducing the emotional impact.

But you can also partially mask the sound of your tinnitus with Brainwave Entrainment audio, rather than music or ambient noise, while you practice tinnitus meditation. It's an incredibly powerful technique that has been used successfully to treat tinnitus in the past. In the course of my research, I came across a 2010 study published in *The Hearing Journal*, which used Binaural Beats rather than white noise, in conjunction with Tinnitus Retraining Therapy protocols, to treat tinnitus patients and help them habituate. Despite its small twenty-six patient sample size, it was a huge success. In a three-month follow-up evaluation, all twenty-six patients reported a reduction in the degree of tinnitus disturbance, with an average reduction of 47.3%. The research methodology also seemed to produce results at a much faster rate than TRT on its own. Yet we can build on this research to achieve even faster and more impactful results, by combining Isochronic Tones (the newer, more powerful iteration of Brainwave Entrainment), partial masking, and tinnitus meditation, all at the same time.

Again, finding the right volume balance between your tinnitus and the audio can be tricky. This is especially true because you'll need to be able to hear the Brainwave Entrainment audio clearly for it to have an effect. But once you get the volume right, and use a high-quality Brainwave Entrainment audio track embedded with the frequencies that correspond with deep meditation, it's magic, especially early on. It enables you to experience a much deeper meditative state, automatically and right from the very start. And because you will be focusing on the sound of your tinnitus while this is happening, your brain will immediately start to associate the deep relaxation of the induced meditative state with the sound of your tinnitus. Of course, if you were just to practice the basic tinnitus meditation technique, this association would still occur. But adding Brainwave Entrainment is like pouring gasoline on a fire. It supercharges the whole process, allowing for much faster progress when you are first starting out.

I have produced a variety of sound masking tracks for this very purpose as part of the Tinnitus Relief Project. You can find them all at Rewiringtinnitus.com/relief.

## Advanced Tinnitus Meditation

All the tools and techniques in this chapter have focused on making tinnitus meditation more effective, and easier to practice, especially when you're just starting out. But as I mentioned before, continually challenging yourself is a crucial part of the overall strategy.

Regardless of whether or not you choose to take

advantage of Brainwave Entrainment and partial masking while practicing tinnitus meditation, you will most likely begin to see preliminary results fairly quickly. As your tinnitus improves, I encourage you to challenge yourself one final time. This last technique will crank up the difficulty level, but if you can master it, you will experience a whole new level of relief. It's a simple technique, but it is not easy.

All you have to do is wear earplugs, and practice tinnitus meditation in total silence. When you practice tinnitus meditation in a quiet room, there is still almost always some level of background noise. Maybe it's the faint hum of your air conditioner or the wind rustling in the trees outside your window. You won't realize how much of a difference this ambient noise makes until you try tinnitus meditation with earplugs for the first time. Earplugs block out everything and eliminate all distractions. It's just you and your tinnitus at full volume. I know that if you are just starting out, this may sound terrifying. I also know that if you are hearing impaired, this may very well resemble your starting point. But practicing tinnitus meditation with earplugs is like working out with a weighted vest. You may struggle initially, but you'll adjust as you get stronger. And when you take the metaphorical vest off, you will feel as light as a feather.

Without question, this is the most difficult thing you can try to do to habituate to the sound of your tinnitus. And while it's not entirely necessary (you can reach the point of full habituation without ever trying this final technique), I recommend you try it at least once when you feel ready. When I was successfully able to meditate to the sound of my tinnitus in total silence, it felt like a huge weight had been lifted off my shoulders. It was my final relief. It was the moment that I knew my tinnitus would no longer bother me, and that should it ever spike, or change, whether in sound or intensity, I would be able to deal with it, and habituate again.

# Part 3:

# Living your Best Life

# with Tinnitus

# Chapter 7

# Better than Before

"Never forget: This very moment, we can change our lives. There never was a moment, and never will be, when we are without the power to alter our destiny."

- Steven Pressfield, author

Up until this point, the strategy has focused on education, and specific techniques designed to enable and speed up the process of habituation. But there is a lot more you can do to improve the quality of your life with tinnitus. Habituation is the answer, but it's not the whole answer. I've mentioned time and again that your tinnitus won't go away, but it will stop bothering you. This is still true. Yet there are countless other things that you can do to further improve your tinnitus.

I will first teach you how to identify your triggers. Regardless of how you ended up with tinnitus, there are most likely specific things that make it worse. These are called triggers, and while many of them are common, each case of tinnitus is unique. Finding the triggers that make your tinnitus worse, and avoiding them, at least initially, will help to speed up your progress. It will also give you the information you need to make better choices for your health.

We will go on to take a look at one of the biggest threats to your continuing success: preventable noise-induced hearing loss. If your tinnitus gets a lot worse or changes in some significant way, you may have to habituate to the sound all over again. In my experience, this isn't necessarily a huge deal. It's easier the second time around, especially if you have continued to practice tinnitus meditation. But it's a better idea to prevent your tinnitus from getting worse in the first place. Preventing noise-induced hearing loss will be of the utmost importance. I will explain why it's such a threat, what to watch out for, and how you can protect your hearing.

After that, we will explore strategies for stress management. Stress can, and will, make your tinnitus considerably worse. Keeping your stress levels under control will be an important part of your tinnitus treatment strategy. Practicing tinnitus meditation is a big step in this direction, but there are a lot of other helpful things you can do as well. I will cover these in detail.

Finally, I will teach you how to get better sleep.

Tinnitus can not only make it hard to fall asleep, but can also severely disrupt the quality. And while your sleep will start to improve as you begin to habituate to the sound, there are steps you can take today that will make a difference.

By the time you finish reading this final section, you will be ready to take on the challenges of tinnitus. This is the final piece of the puzzle. Let's begin.

# Chapter 8

# Finding your Tinnitus Triggers

"Pay attention to the intricate patterns of your existence that you take for granted."

- Doug Dillon, author

## Tracking Tinnitus

W hen you live with tinnitus, the sound isn't always constant. It often fluctuates, and can flare up and get worse for a while. When this happens, it may become a lot louder, and the sound can change. You may hear additional tones or other noises that weren't there before. And while these flare ups and spikes may seem to happen randomly, it's not usually the case. More often than not, spikes are triggered by something external in the environment, or by some problematic aspect of your lifestyle.

There are a wide range of potential triggers, and

everyone reacts differently. What affects other people's tinnitus may not affect yours at all, or may even improve it. There is a huge amount of variance, and without the right approach, it's nearly impossible to figure out what's triggering you. If your tinnitus spikes up at 3 pm because of something you ate for breakfast, you aren't automatically going to make that connection. That's just one example. This sort of missed association happens all the time as most people are just not very good at making these connections naturally. There is, however, an easy way around this shortcoming. A simple practice as old as time: journaling.

When we have the right information in front of us, we're actually very good at finding patterns. Keeping a daily journal will give you the information you need to quickly identify your triggers.

Your journal will serve as a daily record of your tinnitus, and store specific information about your environment and lifestyle. Keeping track of the right variables will enable you to look back and see what was happening on the days your tinnitus was at its worst. Very quickly patterns will emerge, and you will be able to identify your specific triggers. And while you may not be able to actually avoid all of them, it's possible to avoid most of them, which is enough to make a difference.

Journaling can also help you pinpoint the things

that improve your tinnitus, which I like to call wellness triggers. By avoiding your tinnitus triggers, and actively seeking out your wellness triggers, you can give yourself more control over your situation and speed up the time it takes you to improve.

Now let's take a closer look at some of the more common tinnitus triggers.

## Common Tinnitus Triggers

Before I get into the details, I want to mention that there isn't actually any research that specifically links some of these triggers to tinnitus. We don't have all the answers, and a lot more research is still needed. But that also doesn't change the fact that anecdotally most people find that certain activities, foods, supplements, drugs, and environmental factors can cause fluctuations in the sound of their tinnitus.

So we'll start with two of the most common dietary triggers. The first is salt, or more specifically, too much sodium in your diet. It happens to be a major trigger for Meniere's disease, too. But why this seems to be the case for tinnitus is somewhat unclear. Some people believe it has to do with the effect salt can have on blood pressure, others theorize that a high sodium diet can disturb the fluid balance in the inner ear, affecting tinnitus in some way. Salt is a significant trigger for me, but in my opinion, it doesn't matter why. The only thing that matters is what you choose to do about it if you find that too much sodium is a trigger for you, as well. Try reducing your total sodium intake to 1500-2000mg a day, and make sure to space it out evenly over the course of the day.

Caffeine is another common dietary tinnitus trigger. You may find that coffee doesn't affect your tinnitus at all, but if it does, I recommend staying away from it, at least while you're working to habituate. After you habituate, you may find you can tolerate a cup of coffee or two perfectly well. But if it's a trigger for you, avoid it temporarily.

Nicotine, another stimulant, is also a common tinnitus trigger. If you are a smoker, you should consider quitting, and not just to improve your tinnitus, but to reduce the negative impact on your overall health. Electronic cigarettes aren't a good alternative either. With e-cigarettes, you're still consuming nicotine. And the propylene glycol used to make the nicotine liquid has been shown to be ototoxic (toxic to the inner ear) in animals, at least according to one study published in the *American Journal of Otolaryngology* in 1980.

As a former heavy smoker, I know how hard it can be to stop. Ultimately, I was able to quit with nicotine gum. It wasn't easy, but I discovered a few things that helped. When I had a craving for a cigarette, the impulse was to smoke, rather than chew a piece of nicotine gum. The reality, however, was that if I actually chewed a piece of the gum instead, the craving would go away. The trick was to convince myself to chew the gum first. Every time I had a craving, I would tell myself, "If the gum doesn't help in the next ten minutes, I'll have a cigarette." But it always helped, and after about a week, I was able to start weaning off the gum.

Picking a firm quit date is important too. Set a date, tell your family and friends, and stick to it. Your family will be able to help keep you accountable and give you extra encouragement when you need it the most. I know how hard it is to give up smoking, but it's so important.

Alcohol is another common tinnitus trigger. It doesn't seem to affect everyone, but if you discover that it's a trigger for you, I suggest cutting back on your drinking for a little while. At the very least, wait until you have habituated.

Like alcohol, many other recreational drugs are also triggers. I don't condone the use of any illegal recreational drugs, but they are part of our society and need to be acknowledged. When you are first starting out on your journey with tinnitus, I would avoid recreational drugs, especially stimulants, but also any others that seem to worsen your tinnitus.

Allergies and food sensitivities are also triggers for many people. It will be important to find the connections between your allergies and your tinnitus. Journaling can help you identify the patterns, but allergy testing is a good idea as well. It will save you time, and take away the guess work. Try to avoid anything that you know you are allergic to, especially early on. If you happen to be allergic to anything that you can't avoid, such as pollen or dust, you can take a non-drowsy antihistamine like Cetirizine (Zyrtec) during the day. Your doctor may also want to prescribe something stronger if over-the-counter antihistamines are insufficient.

There are also several common environmental tinnitus triggers, some of which will, unfortunately, be entirely outside your control. These can include changes in barometric pressure, certain changes in the weather, pollution, particular types of inflammation in the body, and specific noises and sounds, especially loud ones. If you ever find that your tinnitus is triggered by forces that are outside of your control, or worse, if you can't identify anything specific that's causing the fluctuations in the first place, don't give up hope. You can still focus on the triggers that are within your control, and you will still be able to habituate.

The final common triggers worth noting pertain to lifestyle. Stress and sleep deprivation are big triggers for a lot of people. But they also play a significant role in the quality of your overall health. In the following chapters, I will cover both in detail.

Stress comes in many different shapes and sizes: having an argument with your significant other, working with a manager who breathes down your neck, or having a new child on the way. The list is endless. We can't control most of it either. What we can control is our response to stress. Learning to manage your response to stress will be a crucial part of managing tinnitus.

Sleep is equally important. Getting a full night of quality sleep is one of the best things you can do to improve your health, and your ability to deal with tinnitus. Sleep deprivation, on the other hand, will not only make your tinnitus worse but will also disrupt all other aspects of your health.

If it seems like there are a lot of triggers, don't get discouraged. Remember, everyone experiences tinnitus differently. There is a good chance that only a few of these will actually be a problem for you. It's also not entirely necessary that you avoid your triggers in the first place, you will still eventually be able to habituate. But I do recommend it highly. Discovering your triggers will speed up your progress, lower the intensity of your tinnitus, reduce the number of tinnitus spikes you experience, and will give you some of your power back. It offers you more control over your situation, and enables you to make more informed choices as you go about your life.

# What to Track

I want to be clear, tracking your tinnitus will not be an exact science. The goal is to track the right variables and to look for general trends. With this in mind, here is a list of some of the most helpful data points to log in your journal.

- **Tinnitus Severity**
    - Describe your tinnitus in the morning, afternoon, and evening
        - Volume
        - Intensity
        - Disturbance level
- **Diet**
    - Meals
    - Snacks
    - Total sodium
    - Total sugar

- o   Total water consumption
- o   Caffeine, alcohol, and tobacco
- **Weather**
  - o   Temperature range
  - o   General forecast
  - o   Barometric pressure
  - o   Pollen count
- **Medications**
  - o   Prescription and over-the-counter
    - ▪   Time taken and dosage
  - o   Supplements and vitamins
    - ▪   Time taken and dosage
- **Noise Exposure**
  - o   Have you been exposed to loud sounds?
    - ▪   At what volume level and for how long?
  - o   Did you listen to music with headphones?
    - ▪   At what volume level and for how long?
- **Exercise**
  - o   Type and duration
- **Sleep**
  - o   What time you woke up
  - o   What time you went to bed
  - o   The quality of your sleep

- **Stress**
    - How stressed out are you?
    - What is causing you stress?
    - Did you meditate, and for how long?

To make it as easy as possible for you, I created a one-page PDF journal tool to help you keep track of all the right things.

Get your free copy at Rewiringtinnitus.com/journal.

# Chapter 9

# Protecting your Ears

"One thing I'd tell my younger self - tinnitus is a lot less cool than wearing earplugs."

- Anne Savage, DJ

## How Sound Can Damage our Hearing

Would you willingly destroy your sense of hearing? Would anyone? Of course, the answer is no, but the data seems to tell a different story. Preventable, noise-induced hearing loss is rising to levels we've never seen before. Rock stars are retiring and who can blame them? Record numbers of musicians are developing tinnitus. Some are even finding themselves faced with the choice of retirement or going deaf. And teens are experiencing hearing loss in record numbers too. In fact, they've been hit the hardest of all.

So what's happening here? Why are we suddenly facing an unprecedented epidemic of hearing loss? There are multiple factors, but ultimately it's because we're unwittingly exposing ourselves to dangerously loud levels of sound more often than we ever have before. For the average person, it's a cause for concern. But when you already suffer from tinnitus, or any chronic illness that affects your hearing, it's a wake-up call. We have to take steps to protect our hearing before it's too late.

Many people don't realize that exposure to loud sounds, even for short periods of time, can damage their hearing. When an average healthy hearing person is exposed to loud noise, they will temporarily experience tinnitus and hearing loss. But when you have tinnitus to begin with, it can become much louder. You hope it's only temporary, but that's not always the case. The actual degree of permanent damage will vary depending on the volume and length of exposure. In most instances it will probably be negligible, but the damage is cumulative. Over time, and with repeated exposure, you will start to experience permanent hearing loss. And even a slight increase in hearing loss can cause major changes in the sound of your tinnitus. To understand how sound can do so much damage, we need to take another look at the anatomy of the inner ear.

Here's a quick refresher: Sound waves first enter

through the ear canal, and hit the eardrum, which then sends the sound as vibrations to the middle ear. Next, the three tiny bones of the middle ear, the anvil, hammer, and stirrup, translate these vibrations into physical waves that ripple through the fluid-filled cochlea in the inner ear. Inside the cochlea, microscopic sensory organs called hair cells transform these waves into the electrical signals our brain can understand.

When we perceive sound at a comfortable volume, everything runs smoothly. But as soon as the volume increases past 85 decibels, problems occur. Hearing loss happens when high decibel sounds create violent waves in the delicate fluid of the cochlea, waves that are strong enough to damage the hair cells. The good news is that your hair cells can heal themselves to some extent. It's why noise-induced hearing loss and tinnitus are often temporary, but the hair cells can't keep regenerating indefinitely. Over time, and with repeated exposure to loud sounds, the hair cells will start to die off and leave you with permanent hearing loss.

Unfortunately, as I write this, there is still no way to regenerate these hair cells once they're gone. But there is a great deal of promising research looking to change that. Teams of researchers all over the world are looking at exciting new medical technologies, including gene therapy and stem-cell therapy, to solve this problem.

Many experts expect this to become a reality in the near future. But for the time being, hearing is essentially a limited resource and we can only absorb so many loud sounds before it starts to diminish. When you have tinnitus, or if you have already experienced hearing loss to any degree, you're starting with a disadvantage and need to take action to prevent further damage. You don't want your tinnitus to get worse, and you certainly don't want to lose your sense of hearing.

## Problematic Volume

The first thing that you need to know is that sound is measured in decibels, and 85 decibels is the danger threshold according to the National Institute on Deafness and Other Communication Disorders (NIDCD). Listening to sound at 75 decibels or lower, even for extended periods of time, will not cause permanent damage. But anything from 85 decibels and up will. In fact, if a sound is loud enough, it can immediately cause permanent damage to your hearing. But even when the loss is temporary, you're still causing some degree of permanent damage. Don't forget, your hearing is a finite resource. Once your hair cells die off, there is no going back. Repeated loud sound exposure will lead to hearing loss in the long run, 100% of the time.

To give you an idea of what is safe and what isn't, here are the decibel ratings for several common sounds.

- A whisper – 20 decibels
- The humming of a refrigerator – 45 decibels
- Normal conversation – 60 decibels
- Noise from heavy city traffic – 85 decibels
- Motorcycles – 95 decibels
- An MP3 player at maximum volume – 105-120 decibels

120 Decibels is the average human pain threshold. Anything above this point is going to inflict some degree of physical pain.

Also, our perception of sound is logarithmic. In simple terms, this means that a 20 decibel increase in volume is going to seem roughly four times louder. So a 40 decibel sound is going to seem four times louder than a 20 decibel sound, and a 110 decibel sound is going to seem about 32 times louder than a 60 decibel sound.

- Rock concerts, live music, sports events – 108-130 decibels
- An ambulance siren – 120 decibels
- Thunderclap – 120 decibels
- A jet engine at takeoff – 140 decibels

- Firecrackers and firearms – 150 decibels
- A 12-gauge shotgun – 165 decibels
- A rocket launch – 180 decibels

The rise of smartphones and ear bud headphones is another factor to consider. I mentioned that teens were being hit the hardest. In 2010, a study was published in *The Journal of the American Medical Association* showing a 32% increase in hearing loss among American teens over the previous decade. According to the study, one in five teens in America now suffers from some degree of hearing loss. The problem seems to stem from a lack of understanding. In a World Health Organization (WHO) report, Dr. Etienne Krug, the WHO's Director of the Department for Management of Noncommunicable Diseases, explains, "As they go about their daily lives doing what they enjoy, more and more young people are placing themselves at risk of hearing loss. They should be aware that once you lose your hearing, it won't come back."

Fortunately, we can do something about this. Noise-induced hearing loss is entirely preventable. And if it's what caused your tinnitus in the first place, you can take steps to protect yourself against further damage.

# How to Protect Yourself

There are a lot of effective measures we can take to prevent noise-induced hearing loss. And because hearing loss is permanent, the best offense is a good defense. It's better to be proactive, rather than reactive, and take steps to avoid damage before it happens.

## Be more aware of your sound environment:

Knowing when the noise level is too loud is half the battle. It gives you options. A good rule of thumb is if you think a sound is too loud, it probably is. You can download a free decibel meter app for your smartphone, but keep in mind that it won't be perfectly accurate as the microphone on your phone was not designed for this purpose. It can, however, give you a sense of the ambient volume level, at least up to a certain point. (Sound Meter for Android) (Decibel 10th: Professional Noise Meter for IOS).

## Turn down the volume of your music:

Most headphones and music players can crank out up to 120 decibels or more, the same damaging level as a loud concert. In an article from the American

Osteopathic Association titled "*Hearing Loss and Headphones - Is Anyone Listening?*" Dr. Foy, an osteopathic pediatrician and expert in child hearing loss, offers this suggestion, "If you can't hear anything going on around you when listening to headphones, the decibel level is too high." Dr. Foy suggests listening to music with the volume level at 60%.

## Choose the right kind of headphones:

The type of headphones you use will also make a difference. Over the ear headphones are a better choice than ear buds because the speaker is farther from the eardrum. The problem with ear buds is that they sit very close to the eardrum and create an airtight seal in the ear canal, increasing the intensity and volume of the sound. Over the ear headphones are a much better choice. But nothing is better than over the ear noise-canceling headphones. Because noise-canceling headphones can actively reduce background noise, you can enjoy your music at lower volume levels without a loss in quality.

## Earplugs:

Earplugs are a tried and true method for protecting your ears in loud environments. The type you choose is mostly a matter of personal preference. I prefer the silicone kind, but they all work well when used appropriately. Just make sure you get the correct size, and insert them properly.

## High-Fidelity (Musicians) earplugs:

If you are going to be in a loud environment for an extended period of time, wearing earplugs is a must. The problem is that regular earplugs dampen the sound and make it hard to carry on conversations. If you're at a concert, they will muffle and distort the quality of the music. High-fidelity (musicians) earplugs solve both of these problems by reducing the decibel level of sound without disturbing the quality. If you've never tried these before, they're game changers, and you can find a decent set for as little as $13. A simple search for "Musicians Earplugs" or "High-Fidelity Earplugs" on Amazon or Google will turn up plenty of results. You can even have a custom made pair molded to the unique shape of your ears, although it's much more expensive. My current favorites are ER20 ETY-Plugs made by Etymotic Research and Eargasm Earplugs made by Strand Industries. They are both comfortable, inexpensive and well made. You can find links to all of my favorite earplugs at Rewiringtinnitus.com/bookresources.

Looking back on my life, I wish I had known more about noise-induced hearing loss when I was younger. I know I did a lot of damage to my ears. I constantly listened to loud music with headphones and went to quite a few rock concerts. But living with tinnitus and Meniere's disease has given me a whole new appreciation for my hearing. I had never even considered hearing loss as something I might have to deal with until the day I was diagnosed. My hearing is still good, but I know that could change, and I worry that the damage I did in my teens will catch up with me one day.

Our hearing is such a precious resource, but it's one I took for granted for far too long. Today I'm taking action to keep it, and to prevent my tinnitus from getting worse for as long as I possibly can. I hope you will do the same and protect your hearing before it's too late. You will always be able to re-habituate to the sound of your tinnitus if it does get worse, but it's far easier not to have to in the first place.

# Chapter 10

# Stress Management

"Stress is the trash of modern life - we all generate it, but if you don't dispose of it properly, it will pile up and overtake your life."

- Danzae Pace, author

## Stress and Tinnitus

Depending on whom you ask, there are quite a few things that can exacerbate tinnitus. Everyone seems to have different triggers. But stress happens to be one of the worst and is by far the most common. Even when you fully habituate to the sound of your tinnitus, if your stress levels go up, it can start to bother you again. Eliminating stress wherever possible will play a big role in improving your tinnitus.

So the question is why? Why does stress make our tinnitus so much worse? There are a lot of factors, but it ultimately boils down to several key issues, the first of which has to do with the destructive nature of chronic stress.

We all experience stress in one form or another. It's a fundamental part of life, and we evolved a stress response for a good reason. When faced with danger, we needed to be able to react quickly. Humans may be at the top of the food chain today, but it's not because of our physical strength. Throughout history, most predatory animals could quickly overpower us. It's our brain, our capacity to think, that gives us our great advantage. So to deal with environmental threats, we evolved the fight or flight response to quickly prime the body to respond to danger.

We no longer face the same physical threats as our ancestors, but the stress response remains. The problem is that in today's modern world, threats aren't always clearly defined, and our brains can't distinguish between a perceived threat and real danger. Typically, when our fight or flight response has been activated, and the danger has been resolved, our parasympathetic nervous system kicks in to calm us down and bring us back to baseline. But when the source of the stress is undefined or doesn't go away, we can end up in a state of perpetual arousal and agitation. In small doses, this kind of stress isn't a problem - it's actually a good thing. It provides us with novelty, challenges, and opportunities for growth.

But chronic stress has a profoundly negative effect on our health and is a major trigger for tinnitus. Remember, in fight or flight mode your senses are heightened. Even if you've already habituated, this heightened sense of hearing will make your tinnitus seem louder.

The other issue with stress is that it often finds its way into our physical bodies as muscle tension, aches, and pains. When physical tension spreads into our facial muscles, especially those around the jaw, tinnitus can become much louder. This doesn't happen for everyone, but it's extremely common. If you try clenching your jaw or tensing the muscles around your jaw, you'll see what I mean. Why this happens is still somewhat unclear, but scientists are starting to unravel the mystery. When you clench your jaw, you are manipulating and stimulating specific nerves that project to the dorsal cochlear nucleus (DCN), the part of the brain that helps you locate where a specific sound is coming from. Many scientists believe that this just might be where tinnitus first arises in the brain. A 2012 study published in the journal *Brain Research* analyzed the existing research data and found evidence that supports the theory, or at least shows that the DCN is involved with tinnitus in some capacity.

But at the end of the day, understanding the

connection between tinnitus and stress is less important than knowing how to deal with it. In the remaining part of this chapter, we will explore several powerful strategies, as well as specific techniques, for managing stress.

## Counseling and Therapy

Living with tinnitus can be traumatic, especially if you have suffered for a long period of time. The hopeless despair and seemingly endless torture that so many of us have to endure is enough to leave deep emotional scars. The resulting trauma needs to be addressed. I have experienced the damage first-hand that unresolved trauma can cause. I've witnessed the chaos and devastation that can manifest years after the trauma occurred. Fortunately, there are several good ways to address this problem, sooner rather than later.

I've always had issues with anxiety, but it wasn't really a problem until one of my closest friends unexpectedly passed away when I was 18 years old. Suddenly, my baseline level of anxiety went through the roof. I started having panic attacks, and as the years went on, they got worse. I realize now that I had never properly grieved. If I'm being honest, I didn't really do anything at all to process the death of my friend. The emotions were still bottled up inside of me, and I would lash out at innocent bystanders, leaving a path of destruction in my wake. But at the time, I didn't understand what was happening. It wasn't until much later, in therapy, that the connection between the trauma and my anxiety became clear.

Counseling, or "talk therapy," can be a cathartic and overwhelmingly positive experience when at its best. But just as you need the right doctor to treat your tinnitus, you'll need to find the right therapist, and a therapeutic style that works for you. For me, Cognitive Behavioral Therapy is what worked best. I suspect, however, that my success has had more to do with my actual therapist than the type of therapy. When I was diagnosed with Meniere's disease, I had already been with my therapist for a while, working through my anxiety. His personality really seemed to mesh with mine, and he was always positive, encouraging, and hopeful.

Like most people, he had heard of tinnitus, but not Meniere's disease. Yet he took the time to listen and learn more. He showed me how to stay calm and in the moment when it felt like my world was falling apart. He helped me to process the crazy array of emotions and psychological turmoil that I was experiencing at the time. If you can find a therapist you trust, it can be a powerfully rewarding experience. I also want to point out that while addressing trauma is important, therapy is also an excellent strategy for dealing with stress. A good therapist can help you work through your problems, enabling you to make better decisions. He or she will also be able to help you cope with the emotions and difficulties of treating your tinnitus.

If you're opposed to therapy, or it doesn't fit within your budget, you still have options. Support groups can help as well, albeit in a less professional capacity. Both the American Tinnitus Association and the British Tinnitus Association feature a local support group directory on their websites. I encourage you to take a look as there might be a support group meeting close to where you live. Otherwise, there are many vibrant support communities online. Having a place to openly vent frustrations, celebrate successes, and communicate with others in the same situation can be extremely helpful. There are forums and message boards solely devoted to tinnitus with large numbers of active participants. You can also find several great support groups on Facebook, some with thousands of members. Questions are usually answered very quickly and by a wide variety of people with different backgrounds and experiences. A list of online support communities can be found in the resources section in the back of this book.

These groups can be a fantastic resource, but I have to warn you, if you find that spending time in these communities to be depressing, I suggest you avoid them for a while. Some of the groups can occasionally have a "misery loves company" kind of feel. If a group is putting a damper on your mood in any way, it's better to explore other, more positive avenues. There is always so much hope. Never forget that.

# Physical Stress Management

Managing the mental side of stress is important, but it's only one part of the equation. You also need to pay attention to your body. Stress has a tendency to work its way into our physical bodies as tension, knots, physical aches and pains, and general discomfort. Reducing the stress in your body will not only help you feel more relaxed but will benefit you mentally and emotionally, as well. The mind and body are intimately connected, and taking a whole body, or holistic, approach to your health is a better way to manage stress. It can have a powerful impact on your tinnitus.

## Massage:

Massage, in all its forms, may seem like a luxury, but it's a powerful tool for healing. An experienced masseuse can relieve tense and knotted muscles throughout the entire body. We tend to store anxiety, stress, emotional pain, and fear as physical tension in the body. It's an insidious type of tension too. We don't even realize the toll it's taking on us until it gets so bad that we feel it as pain. Getting a professional massage once a month has had a transformative effect on my stress levels. It's mind- boggling how much tension accumulates in my muscles over the course of a single month. If you can afford it, getting a massage, even if it's only once every couple of months, can be extremely effective for dealing with stress.

If a professional massage is not in the budget, there are additional, less expensive ways of reducing physical tension. My personal favorite also happens to be the least expensive option: the lacrosse ball. You can find them at any sporting goods store for a couple of dollars, and they can be used to massage and work the tension out of most of the muscles in your body. Generally, I will lie on my back with the lacrosse ball under my shoulder blades and slowly work the ball around my back and shoulder muscles. It works really well on sore feet too. Be gentle at first, and slowly add pressure as needed. A simple Google search for "lacrosse ball massage" will bring up thousands of instructional videos and articles.

## Acupuncture:

Acupuncture is one of the main components of Traditional Chinese Medicine (TCM) and is a practice that dates back thousands of years. To understand acupuncture, you must first understand that TCM is founded on the belief that the body contains a system of energy flow pathways called meridians. Hundreds of points, called meridian points, have been identified along these pathways and are believed to have a direct effect on the body. The energy that flows through the meridian pathways is known as Qi (pronounced chi). TCM follows the thinking that our health is closely tied to the free flow of Qi and that blockages result in health problems. An acupuncturist places long, thin needles into various meridian points to clear these blockages.

I know it sounds esoteric, but I encourage you to keep an open mind. In the last decade, Western culture has seen a massive rise in the popularity of acupuncture as a means to treat a wide variety of ailments, illnesses, and pain. Many hospitals now offer therapeutic acupuncture as an accompaniment to pharmaceutical and traditional medical interventions. It also happens to be extremely effective at managing stress. And interestingly enough, some tinnitus patients even report improvement after a series of targeted acupuncture sessions. At the very least, give it a try before you make a judgment. TCM has existed far longer than our Western, science-based medicine. Its longevity is a testament to its efficacy.

When I was first diagnosed with Meniere's disease, I immediately started seeing an acupuncturist. It definitely lessened my vertigo and seemed to help me cope with my tinnitus, too. Some people experience immediate results from acupuncture, while for others it may take several sessions, if it works at all. But it's important to find an experienced acupuncturist for the best chance of success. A quick Google search should reveal several in your area. Call and talk to them, and don't be afraid to ask questions. Find out if they have treated patients with tinnitus before. I was surprised to find that my acupuncturist had treated Meniere's patients, as well as patients with other causes of vertigo and tinnitus.

### Saunas:

Saunas are not only another fantastic tool for physical stress reduction but can also help to increase your overall capacity for managing stress. The intense heat quickly relaxes sore and stiff muscles, and leaves you feeling fantastic. Twenty minutes in the sauna should be more than enough to work up a good sweat. I always feel deeply relaxed and refreshed after I come out of the sauna, especially if I got a good workout in beforehand. Just remember to stay hydrated. Drink plenty of water before you go into the sauna and once you've finished.

# Exercise

The importance of exercise goes well beyond its ability to help you manage stress. It has a powerful effect on your wellbeing and is an integral part of being healthy. Adding exercise to your daily routine, even in the smallest amounts, can offer tremendous benefits at every level of your progress with tinnitus. For starters, an exercise practice will improve all other aspects of your physical health, which can help to speed up the time it takes you to habituate. It will also reduce your stress levels, improve the quality and duration of your sleep, and help you build momentum in your treatment efforts. Depending on your level of fitness, you may not be able to hit the gym and start lifting weights, but you still have plenty of options. Let's take a look at several good ways to approach exercise.

## Walking:

Exercise does not have to be intense to reap the benefits. In fact, if you are not physically ready for intense exercise, it can be a detriment. If you aren't in the best physical shape, start slowly and take your time in building up to a more complete exercise routine.

One of the easiest ways to get started is just to go for a walk. That's all it takes for your brain to start releasing endorphins, your body's "feel good" chemicals. Ever hear someone refer to a runner's high? They're talking about endorphins, which cause stress levels to go down and overall feelings of satisfaction to go up. If you feel depressed or stressed out, the endorphins released during exercise can help to lift your spirits.

If you are new to exercise, I recommend you find a way to add walking to your daily routine. And for an added bonus, avoid the treadmill and go for a walk outside. It's much more enjoyable, especially when the weather is nice. Eventually, you can build on this and start adding intensity and complexity to your routine, but it's not necessary, especially early on. When starting out, your goal should just be to get yourself up and moving, for a period of time, every single day.

## Cardio:

If you are in reasonably good shape or ready for a more difficult form of exercise, a good cardiovascular workout is a wonderful way to improve your health and drastically lower stress levels. It's hard to put into words how good I feel after a really intense run. The mental clarity, feeling of accomplishment, and almost euphoric sense of well-being is beyond compare. It's also an effective way to get in shape. Personally, I love to run, but I also enjoy riding my bike. I'll get on the elliptical from time to time as well, just to mix things up. There are countless ways to get a good cardio workout, so rather than attempting to cover each one, I'll give you a few helpful guidelines to follow.

I recommend starting out slowly. Always warm up for five to ten minutes before you increase the intensity. You can hurt yourself by trying to go too fast, or turning up the resistance too quickly. Increase the level of difficulty slowly, and over time, for the best results. Your body will thank you for it. Also, taking your workout outside can make it much more enjoyable. Running or jogging in a beautiful park or through a big city can add an element of novelty and excitement to the experience. The sunlight and fresh air can keep you happy and motivated in a way that generally isn't found at the gym.

And the ambient noise can help to mask the sound of your tinnitus. Going for a bike ride outdoors is always a lot of fun too, especially with friends. But regardless of what you choose to do, make sure you stay hydrated, and aim for at least twenty minutes of cardio.

## Yoga:

Yoga is another effective way to add exercise into your routine with specific benefits for someone with tinnitus. In many ways, it's the perfect exercise for anyone trying to habituate. It combines elements of exercise with meditation, breath control, stretching, and balance. The meditative aspects of yoga help to reduce stress, while the practice of breath control promotes an improvement in emotional stability and a sense of calm in the face of adversity. All of these elements will help you to improve your tinnitus meditation practice and your emotional response to the sound. It's a powerful weapon against tinnitus.

If you are interested in trying yoga, there are several good ways to get started. The first is to find a local yoga studio and take a beginner's class. There are many different types of yoga, and I recommend trying several styles to find what resonates with you the most. Yogafinder.com is a great resource to search for studios in your area. A simple Google search should also provide a good list of nearby options.

If you don't want to go to a class, there are thousands of instructional yoga videos you can watch in the comfort of your home. Amazon is an excellent resource for this. Through Amazon Video, you can access and stream thousands of different yoga videos. Many of the titles are also available on DVD. Otherwise, you can search YouTube for yoga routines. A search for "Yoga" brings up nearly six million results, and on YouTube, all the yoga videos are free. Plus, many of the videos are only 20-30 minutes long, which is perfect for beginners.

## Personal Training:

I know it can be expensive, but if you're able to afford it, a personal trainer can help you get the most out of your exercise practice. They are one-on-one fitness coaches who will "hold your hand" and guide you through the process of getting in shape. The right trainer can teach you the best exercises, develop routines customized specifically for you and your abilities, and can help you get into shape regardless of your current limitations or skill level. They can set realistic goals, while designing specific workouts and routines to enable you to achieve those goals.

# Tinnitus as a Signal of Health

As you begin to habituate to the sound of your tinnitus, you will eventually start to notice it slip from your awareness. At first, it may only be for short periods of time. But it won't be long before you suddenly find that a day, or even several days, have passed and you haven't thought about your tinnitus once. In his short book, *A Positive Tinnitus Story*, author and tinnitus expert Julian Cowan Hill offers a great analogy, "It's a bit like being able to feel your socks. You can feel them if you really focus, but why would you bother?" Once you fully habituate, the noise will still be there when you consciously look for it, but you won't be thinking about it all the time. And this is where things get interesting.

Having poor health, not getting enough sleep, or eating an unhealthy diet can all contribute to higher stress levels and can make your tinnitus worse. As you habituate, the intensity of your tinnitus can be used as a way to measure the quality of your health. If you find that it's suddenly much louder, there is likely something going on with your health that needs to be addressed. Julian explains, "Let your tinnitus be a healthometre. If it backs off, you are doing the right things. If it pipes up, then look at what you are experiencing, what you are exposing yourself to, and how you are driving yourself. If you work with your tinnitus, it will guide you back to a healthier life!" Ultimately, this is just one more way your tinnitus can be used as something positive. The more you can make the sound work for you, the faster you can habituate.

On its own, tinnitus meditation is a powerful tool for relieving stress, but many of the techniques I've covered in this chapter will help you go the extra mile. When you have lived with severe tinnitus for a long time, it can take a lot of effort to get the ball rolling in the right direction. The more tools you have at your disposal, the better off you'll be.

In addition to stress, many people with tinnitus also struggle with their sleep. The constant noise can make it seem impossible to get the deep restorative sleep you need to feel better. But there are things you can start to do today to change that. In the next chapter, I will teach you not only how to fall asleep faster, but how to get deeper, longer, and higher-quality sleep, as well.

# Chapter 11

# Getting Better Sleep

"The worst thing in the world is to try to sleep and not to."

- F. Scott Fitzgerald, author

## Sleep Deprivation and Tinnitus

In the early days of my Meniere's disease diagnosis, my tinnitus got significantly worse, and my sleep really started to suffer. Falling asleep is a big challenge for most people with tinnitus. We try to ignore it, or to block it out with background noise, but the harder we try, the worse it can get. When faced with such a difficult situation, a lot of people turn to sleeping pills or alcohol, and who can blame them? But it doesn't solve anything. In fact, it can lead to even more problems down the road, and both can disrupt the quality of your sleep. Regardless of how you have chosen to deal with this issue in the past, sleep deprivation can have devastating consequences. Even for the average healthy adult, the effects are debilitating. But when you have tinnitus, chronic sleep deprivation can crank up your stress levels and make your tinnitus considerably worse. It can quickly unwind any progress you may have made.

It's important to understand that your body does not treat sleep like a bank. You can't save up sleep and try to go for days without it. You also can't "overdraft" without consequences, getting less sleep during the week and expecting just to make it up on the weekends. To actually get the benefits that sleep provides for your health, you have to make an effort to get high-quality sleep as often as possible.

In the short term, sleep deprivation will reduce your cognitive performance and alertness, even after just one night of poor sleep. It will start to affect your memory too. Lack of sleep can also decrease your ability to handle stress, while at the same time increasing your overall stress load. It will depress your immune system and may increase levels of inflammation throughout your body.

But the long-term effects of chronic sleep deprivation are even worse: high blood pressure, higher risk of heart attack and heart failure, higher risk of stroke, obesity, mental health issues such as anxiety disorders and depression, attention disorders such as ADD, a decrease in emotional intelligence, and an overall reduction in quality of life. I find that when I don't get enough sleep for several days in a row, my health starts to break down, my tinnitus gets much louder, and my Meniere's symptoms flare up.

Tinnitus meditation and the other techniques you have learned can help you to improve your sleep. But they all take time to start working, and during that time, the effects of sleep deprivation can dramatically slow your progress. The best thing you can do, starting tonight, is take specific actions to improve your sleep. It will act as a force multiplier that enhances all of your other efforts, making them more effective.

## Upgrade your Sleep Routine

Many people, regardless of whether they have tinnitus or not, don't have a very good pre-sleep routine. In their defense, it's probably not intentional. They just don't know any better, and there are so many different variables that can affect the quality of sleep. Fortunately, most of them are easy to learn, and once you understand what's affecting you, you can make the changes necessary to start benefiting immediately.

## Use routines to your advantage:

The problem a lot of people run into is they don't actually have a sleep routine of any kind in the first place. Either that, or they have one that isn't helpful. But following a routine that promotes a more restful night's sleep can be extremely beneficial. It can help you fall asleep faster, and get better sleep, more consistently.

The first step is to keep regular sleeping hours. If you are going to bed and waking up at different times every day, it can put you in a state similar to jet lag and prevent you from getting the deep restorative sleep you need. Get yourself on a schedule. Go to sleep and wake up at the same time every single day. Also, keep in mind that throughout the night, the nature of sleep changes in a regular and predictable way. There are several phases of sleep, each serving a different purpose, that occur in repeating 90-minute cycles. Each cycle includes a period of physiologically restorative deep sleep, a transition to lighter sleep, and psychologically restorative REM (rapid eye movement) sleep, where our minds are highly active, and dreaming occurs.

Most people sleep through four to six 90-minute sleep cycles each night, for a total of six to nine hours. If you find you're often tired in the morning, you can try this simple trick to wake up with more energy. Just set your alarm to correspond with the end of a sleep cycle. In other words, rather than the standard eight hours of sleep, get seven and a half or nine hours instead. You can always change your sleep schedule later on if you need to, but for now, and at least until you have habituated to the sound of your tinnitus, stick to a schedule.

Once you have adjusted your sleeping hours, the next step is to follow a fixed routine, every single night, before you go to bed. What you choose to do during this time matters, but not as much as being consistent. If you do the same things every single night before you go to bed, your brain will quickly start to associate your routine with falling asleep. Pretty soon, the routine alone will be enough to make you start yawning.

## Turn off all screens 90 minutes before bedtime:

For better or worse, bright backlit screens have come to dominate our lives. Our smartphones, tablets, laptops, and TVs have become the centerpieces of our increasingly interconnected world. They enhance our lives in numerous ways, but they also disrupt the quality of our sleep.

Our bodies maintain an internal day/night cycle known as the circadian rhythm. During the day, sunlight triggers our bodies to secrete daytime hormones. Later, in the absence of sunlight, our brains secrete a hormone called melatonin that lets our bodies know that it's time to get ready to go to sleep. Unfortunately, the bright blue light spectrum emitted from our various screens mimics sunlight, and causes the brain to shut down melatonin production. Watching TV, reading on an iPad, or playing games on a phone before going to bed, can make it much harder to fall asleep. It can also degrade the quality of your sleep.

To avoid this, you have several options. The best thing you can do is simply to turn off all backlit screens 90 minutes before bedtime. Read a book (a paper book, not an eBook) instead or spend time with loved ones. It's the best way to ensure a good night's sleep. But you can also take steps to block out the blue light spectrum from your devices. There are two good ways to do this. You can purchase a pair of special glasses that block the blue light spectrum, or you can get an app to do it for you. With the glasses, the price depends on the style. You can find reasonably priced glasses and clip-on lenses on Amazon.com or you can opt for more expensive alternatives such as the famous Blublocker brand. (Visit Rewiringtinnitus.com/bookresources for a complete list) Otherwise, you can install an app on your mobile devices and computers to dim the screen, and apply a red filter that turns off most of the blue light spectrum. (F.Lux for Computers) (Twilight for Android Devices) (iOS has this feature built in: Go to Settings > Display & Brightness > Night Shift)

## Perform a mind dump:

When trying to fall asleep, a lot of the mental chatter that people experience stems from trying to juggle a list of things to remember. It's especially bad when you are trying to fall asleep and you suddenly have a good idea. But no matter what thoughts are swirling around in your head, the act of putting them down on paper before you get in bed can really quiet things down.

The best way to do this is to perform what I like to call a mind dump. Grab a pen and a piece of paper and write down anything and everything that's going through your mind. It's as simple as that. You will find that you can fall asleep much more easily when your thoughts and ideas are safely written down. It's also a good way to remember things that are important. Sleep has a strange way of robbing us of our best ideas, no matter how sure we are that we'll remember them in the morning. Most people don't. If you find that you still have persistent thoughts and ideas after your mind dump, turn the light back on and write down anything else you may have missed.

## Cut out the caffeine:

Caffeine is a double-edged sword for people with tinnitus. On the one hand, it can give us a nice boost of energy. But it also makes it very difficult to fall asleep and can affect the quality of our sleep, especially if consumed in the afternoon or evening. It's also a very common tinnitus trigger because caffeine stimulates the nervous system in a big way. When your tinnitus is driving you crazy, your nervous system is already overly activated, and drinking caffeine can strengthen your stress response. It can make it almost impossible to fall asleep.

If you are just starting to work on your tinnitus, I recommend cutting out caffeine entirely. You can always add it back in later on, but for now, stick to decaf. Caffeine can be an obstacle to habituation and removing it can immediately improve the quality of your sleep. At the very least, cut back on your overall caffeine intake and avoid it completely within eight hours of your bedtime.

## Take the right supplements:

Several supplements can help you get a better night's sleep, though none are as important as magnesium. Because most people are deficient, getting extra magnesium into your system can often improve your sleep and lower your stress levels at the same time. In his best-selling book, *Sleep Smarter*, author and health expert Shawn Stevenson explains:

"Magnesium is a bonafide anti-stress mineral. It helps to balance blood sugar, optimize circulation and blood pressure, relax tense muscles, reduce pain, and calm the nervous system. Yet, because it has so many functions, it tends to get depleted from our bodies rather fast. Magnesium deficiency is likely the number one mineral deficiency in our world today. Estimates show that upwards of 80 percent of the population in the United States is deficient in magnesium. And, some experts say that these numbers are actually conservative. Chances are, you're not getting enough magnesium into your system, and getting your magnesium levels up can almost instantly reduce your body's stress load and improve the quality of your sleep."

There are several ways you can boost your magnesium levels. The first is through direct supplementation, but not all magnesium supplements are created equal. You want to make sure you take the right form. Look for magnesium aspartate, malate, glycinate, threonate, or orotate. These forms have higher absorption rates and are far more effective. Take 400-800 mg of magnesium daily.

Transdermal magnesium supplements are also an excellent choice as magnesium absorbs through the skin incredibly well. Taking a bath with Epsom salts, which are loaded with magnesium, is one option. Another is to apply magnesium skin creams. Look for pharmaceutical grade skin creams containing magnesium chloride hexahydrate.

A quick word of caution though. Magnesium supplements should not be taken by anyone with compromised kidney function. They also should not be taken with calcium supplements or dairy products, as magnesium can interfere with calcium absorption. Lastly, magnesium supplements can interfere with the effectiveness of other medications, including blood pressure medications, so **make sure to speak with your doctor first**.

In addition to magnesium, there are several other natural herbal sleep aids that are worth mentioning. Chamomile tea, for example, is an extremely effective and popular choice. It can safely induce sleep, is healthy for you, and is not addictive. Valerian root is good too.

It's a powerful herbal sedative that can help you fall asleep when chamomile tea isn't strong enough. Both are available in most nutrition and convenience stores.

Supplemental melatonin can be taken as a sleep aid, too. But always exercise caution and only use it as a short-term solution. Melatonin is a hormone and should be treated as such. If used only occasionally, it can work fantastically well. (It can also help avoid jet lag by resetting your body's circadian rhythm when traveling across time zones). It should not, however, be used as a long-term solution.

## Brainwave Entrainment for Sleep:

We learned earlier that audio based Brainwave Entrainment can quickly induce a deep state of meditation. Fortunately, it can also be used to help you get to sleep. By synchronizing your brainwave patterns to the frequencies that correspond with falling asleep, you can drift off in a matter of minutes.

I have used Brainwave Entrainment audio for years to help me fall asleep, and have found there to be many benefits. The most obvious of which is its ability to induce sleep without drugs or medication. With prescription sleeping pill use on the rise, and the potentially harmful side effects and complications they can create, any effective solution that can help you fall asleep without chemicals should be explored.

I have created several Brainwave Entrainment tracks specifically designed to help tinnitus sufferers fall asleep faster. You can find them, along with all the other tracks I've created at: Rewiringtinnitus/relief

# Optimize your Sleep Environment

The way your bedroom is set up has an enormous impact on the quality of your sleep. It could be affecting you right now. The good news is that there are several simple changes you can make to your bedroom which will immediately improve the quality of your sleep.

### Make your room pitch black:

If you have a lot of ambient light coming into your bedroom from nightlights, cable boxes, alarm clocks, street lights, or from any other source, it can disturb your sleep. The best strategy is to make your room as dark as possible. You can buy blackout curtains at most department stores that will completely block out any light coming in from the outside. But also make sure to cover every source of light in your bedroom, no matter how small. Ideally, you want the room to be pitch black.

This is something you can do right now to improve the quality of your sleep. If, however, you don't want to make any changes to your bedroom, you can always just wear a sleep mask that covers your eyes. It works really well, though some people may find it uncomfortable.

## The right temperature is colder than you think:

Most people keep the temperature in their bedroom much warmer than it should be. Believe it or not, studies have shown that we actually get the best sleep when the temperature in the room is between 60 and 68 degrees Fahrenheit. It's much cooler than most people would expect and has to do with an internal process called thermoregulation. Again Shawn Stevenson explains, "When it's time for your body to rest, there is an automatic drop in your core body temperature to help initiate sleep. If the temperature in your environment stays too high, then it can be a bit of a physiological challenge for your body to get into the ideal state for restful sleep."

If the temperature is much warmer or cooler than the optimum range, it might impact your sleep. But you also don't want to be cold. You need to feel comfortable under your blankets. So wearing socks is a good option if your feet get cold at this temperature. I find that when

I keep my thermostat at 68 degrees with the ceiling fan on low, I can fall asleep much more easily.

## The sound of your bedroom:

As many of you know by now, sound can have a direct impact on your sleep. For someone with tinnitus, this presents an interesting set of challenges. Normally, it's important to have a silent sleep environment. Even a small noise may be enough to wake you, and whether or not you remember it the next morning is irrelevant. It disrupts your sleep cycles and lowers your quality of sleep. The challenge here is that tinnitus is typically much worse and more noticeable in silence. Once you habituate it won't be a problem, but in the meantime you have a few options. If you still have some of your hearing left, your best bet is to mask the sound of your tinnitus, drowning it out with relaxing background noise. Most of you probably already do this to some extent. The masking sound will not only lower the perceived volume of your tinnitus, which will help you to relax, but it will provide a constant background noise to block out other sounds as well, improving your sleep.

There are hundreds of white noise and ambient sound machines available on Amazon. Some of them are pretty good. But in my opinion, a portable Bluetooth speaker connected to your smartphone is a better choice. It gives you the option to use any sound masking audio tracks you may have downloaded, or one of the thousands of sound therapy apps available for both Android and iOS devices. If your tinnitus is particularly bad, you can even get a soft headband with integrated speakers designed to be worn while lying in bed.

(Visit Rewiringtinnitus.com/bookresources for a full list.)

Yet not everyone will be able to use sound masking to help them fall asleep. Fortunately, you can also use a modified version of the tinnitus meditation technique to transform the sound into a tool for inducing sleep.

## Using Tinnitus to Fall Asleep Faster

Once you have practiced tinnitus meditation successfully several times and have gotten past the initial difficulty, you can use a modified version of the technique to fall asleep. It's incredibly useful and just one more way you can put your tinnitus to work for you.

Part of the reason it works so well is the mentally calming nature of meditation, yet the progressive muscle relaxation plays an important role as well. More often than not, it's physical tension that makes sleep difficult. When you fall asleep, your body and brain go through a series of changes. Your brainwaves slow down, and your body starts to physically relax. But you can hack this process by consciously relaxing your body first. It's amazing how much physical tension we can hold in our muscles without realizing it. It's not until you focus intensely on relaxing muscle groups throughout your body that you start to notice it. Once the tension is released, your body can begin to drop into sleep.

By combining the tinnitus meditation technique with visualization, aspects of self-hypnosis, and trance meditation, I developed a routine that could quickly get me to sleep. You can practice it yourself, but if possible, it's helpful to have someone else guide you through it.

## The Tinnitus Sleep Induction Technique:

Close your eyes and take five deep breaths into your diaphragm (lower abdomen). Feel your stomach expand as you inhale, and with each exhale, feel your entire body becoming more and more relaxed. Let all your muscles go completely limp.

Now focus on individual muscle groups, one at a time, relaxing each as much as possible before moving on. Let all the tension dissolve as you work your way through your body.

Start with your feet and your toes. Let all of the muscles go completely limp. Now focus on your legs and your butt. Release all the tension. Continue on to your stomach and your lower back, then your chest and upper back, your shoulders and your arms, your hands and your fingers, your neck and your throat, and finally, your head and your face.

Take a deep breath. Now that your muscles are completely relaxed, focus your attention on the sound of your tinnitus. Maintain a mindset of curiosity, as if you were observing something interesting for the first time. Continue to breathe naturally and keep your mind focused on the sound. If and when your mind starts to wander, and you notice it, gently bring your focus back to the sound. Do this for several minutes.

Finally, imagine that your bed is inside an elevator that's descending deep underground with the doors still open. Imagine that the elevator shaft is made of dirt and rocks, and as you descend, watch the walls as they appear to be moving up, as your bed sinks deeper and deeper down the elevator shaft. Try to sense the sinking with your entire body. You may be surprised to find that it actually feels like the bed is moving down beneath you. Hold this in your imagination for as long as you can. Feel the bed sinking, down and down and down. Deeper and deeper down. (Mentally repeat, "Down and down and down. Deeper and deeper and deeper down." for as long as you are able.)

By this point, you should be on the verge of falling asleep, or at the very least, deeply relaxed. This technique becomes more effective the more often you practice it. Your body will start to associate the routine with falling asleep.

It's quite helpful to have someone else verbally guide you through the mental imagery of this routine, but I know that won't always be possible. For this reason, I have included guided tinnitus sleep induction tracks as part of the Tinnitus Relief Project at Rewiringtinnitus.com/relief. The first time I tried this with my wife Megan, she was asleep before I could finish. She had been tossing and turning for over an hour. I hope it works for you as well as it has worked for us.

Chapter 12

# Action Plan

"Action may not always bring happiness, but there is no happiness without action."

- Benjamin Disraeli, former British Prime Minister

## Tools and Bonuses

**Tinnitus Trigger Tool (FREE):**
Rewiringtinnitus.com/journal

You should start tracking your tinnitus and your lifestyle right away. It takes time to discover your specific tinnitus triggers, so you'll want to get in the habit of journaling every day, sooner rather than later. Download the Rewiring Tinnitus Trigger Tool PDF and fill one out each day. You can print it and fill it out by hand, or fill it out on the computer and print it out when you are finished. Keep each finished page in a folder.

**The Tinnitus Relief Project Audio Package (Optional):**
Rewiringtinnitus.com/relief

A set of 49 audio tracks engineered to help you find relief from tinnitus either by enhancing all the techniques found in this book. You will not need it to successfully habituate, but if you choose to use it, make sure to download it first and have it set up before you begin. If you have significant hearing loss in both ears, do not download this package, as it is all audio based.

## How to Use the Optional
## Tinnitus  Relief Project Audio Package:

**Sound Masking Audio:** At any point in your treatment, you can use these ambient soundtracks to partially mask the sound of your tinnitus while you practice the techniques. This strategy is adopted from Tinnitus Retraining Therapy. By lowering the perceived volume of your tinnitus, all of the techniques will be easier to implement. You can also use these tracks to mask your tinnitus when you go to sleep.

**Brainwave Entrainment Relaxation Audio:** These Brainwave Entrainment audio tracks are engineered to induce a deep state of relaxation. You can use them to relax and relieve anxiety before attempting any of the techniques. It can drastically reduce your stress and anxiety levels, making the techniques easier to approach. You can also use these tracks for general stress relieving purposes.

**Brainwave Entrainment Meditation Audio:** Think of these Brainwave Entrainment audio tracks as guided meditations that can communicate to your brain. All the meditation tracks are engineered to induce a deep state of meditation for a set period of time. These tracks are designed to be used with tinnitus meditation. Simply set the volume of the track at a level that partially masks the sound of your tinnitus and begin meditating. The track will put you in an advanced meditative state automatically and within minutes. This is the most powerful way to practice tinnitus meditation and it can greatly speed up the habituation process.

**Guided Meditations:** I have also included guided meditations to make your treatment process easier. There are guided meditations with no background audio and meditations layered with Brainwave Entrainment. Simply load the track, set the volume to a level that only partially masks your tinnitus, and follow along.

**Brainwave Entrainment Sleep Inducing Audio:** These tracks are engineered to do one thing and one thing only: get you to sleep. Tinnitus can make it really hard to fall asleep, and insomnia can make your tinnitus worse. These tracks can help you get the sleep you need, especially early on, so that you can start to improve.

**Brainwave Entrainment Focus Enhancing Audio:** When your tinnitus is at its worst, it can be very difficult to stay focused on important tasks. These tracks will boost your mental energy levels and help to keep you focused while masking the sound of your tinnitus at the same time. Simply listen to one of these tracks as you work or any time you need help focusing.

# Practice Schedule

As you set out on your tinnitus treatment journey, I want to give you every possible chance to succeed. I know that I have covered a great deal of information over the course of this book, from theories to research, specific techniques and strategies, and I want to make sure you don't feel overwhelmed.

So to make it easy for you get started, I've included a practice schedule for you to follow for the first week.

## Before you begin:

- Download the Rewiring Tinnitus Trigger Tool (Rewiringtinnitus.com/journal)
- Download the optional Tinnitus Relief Project Audio Package (Rewiringtinnitus.com/relief)

## Keep in mind:

- The suggested time limits for each meditation are only guidelines. If you have previous experience with meditation or are comfortable with the technique, feel free to practice the tinnitus meditation techniques for as long as you like. The shorter time limits are to give you an achievable goal and make it easier for the practice to become a habit. But I've found that longer sessions are incredibly effective.

- You do not have to follow the exact order I've suggested below. All the techniques I've described throughout the book are effective, and you are more than welcome to mix and match as you progress at your own pace. Having said that, the following schedule is designed to work best for people who are new to meditation, or have a more severe case of tinnitus.

# Day 1:

- **Tinnitus Journaling Exercise:** Complete the initial tinnitus journaling exercise. It is an important first step and will give you an opportunity to face your tinnitus in a low-pressure environment.

  o **If your tinnitus is severe, or if you are having a hard time completing this exercise:** Listen to one of the Brainwave Entrainment Relaxation tracks first, and then use ambient noise to partially mask the sound of your tinnitus as you complete the exercise. Doing both will make it easier for you to face your tinnitus for the first time.

- **Basic Tinnitus Meditation Technique (5 minutes):** Even if you have previous meditation experience, I recommend no more than five minutes on your first day. However, if you find that you are comfortable with this right away, feel free to meditate for as long as you like.

  o Optional - listen to one of the Brainwave Entrainment Relaxation tracks first, and use sound masking to partially mask the sound of your tinnitus. Alternatively, you can listen to one of the guided tinnitus meditations with Brainwave Entrainment.

- Fill out a Tinnitus Trigger Tool Journal page

## Day 2:

- **Tinnitus Meditation (5-15 minutes):** Start with the basic technique and once you have found a comfortable rhythm, practice the first variation, and add visualization into the mix.
  - o Optional - either listen to one of the Brainwave Entrainment Relaxation tracks first or use one of the Brainwave Entrainment Meditation tracks during your session.

- Fill out a Tinnitus Trigger Tool Journal page

## Day 3:

- **Tinnitus Meditation (5-15 minutes):** Start with the basic technique and once you have found a comfortable rhythm, practice the first variation again, adding visualization.

- Fill out a Tinnitus Trigger Journal page

## Day 4:

- **Tinnitus Meditation:** Start with the basic technique and once you have found a comfortable rhythm, expand your awareness and practice the second variation to work on your awareness control.

- Fill out a Tinnitus Trigger Journal page

## Day 5:

- **Tinnitus Meditation (5-15 minutes):** Start with the basic technique and once you have found a comfortable rhythm, practice the first variation, adding visualization to your meditation. After several minutes, expand your awareness and practice the second variation to work on your awareness control.

- Fill out a Tinnitus Trigger Journal page

## Day 6:

- **Tinnitus Meditation (5-15 minutes):** Start with the basic technique and once you have found a comfortable rhythm, practice the first variation, adding visualization to your meditation. After several minutes, expand your awareness and practice the second variation to work on your awareness control.

- Fill out a Tinnitus Trigger Journal page

# Day 7:

- **Basic Tinnitus Meditation Technique (10+ minutes):** Practice the basic tinnitus meditation technique only for at least ten minutes.

- Fill out a Tinnitus Trigger Journal page

- **Review your Tinnitus Trigger Journal pages from the past week:** Compare the days when your tinnitus was at its worst and start to look for patterns. Was there anything in common on those days? Make a note of anything you think might be a trigger for you. Also, compare the days when your tinnitus was at its best and look for commonalities. This will be an ongoing process of discovery. Be sure to look back and compare your journal pages periodically.

## Moving forward:

- **Practice Tinnitus Meditation at least once a day:** You can vary the techniques however you'd like. As you get a sense of what works best for you, stick with it.

- **Continue to track your Tinnitus:** The more data you have, the better the chances that you will be able to identify your unique tinnitus triggers.

- **Work to reduce your stress levels**

- **Exercise regularly**

- **Work to increase the quality of your sleep**

# **Conclusion**

"Believe in yourself and all that you are. Know that there is something inside of you that is greater than any obstacle."

- Christian D. Larson, author

Over the years, I've had to face a lot of health-related adversities, but my struggle with tinnitus was uniquely challenging. I was tormented by the sound, day and night, for so long. But I no longer think of it as a bad thing. I now use my tinnitus as a tool to help me meditate, relax, and fall asleep. It lets me know when my stress levels are out of whack and when I need to put more effort into managing my health. I've successfully befriended my torturer. It's a much better way to live.

I'm lucky to have found ways to habituate to my tinnitus. So many people don't. But it is always possible. And that possibility is all the hope you need to get started.

A part of me still wonders what life would be like without tinnitus. Another part of me hopes that one day, science will answer that question. Tinnitus research is picking up at an astounding rate. All over the world, research and studies are underway. Pharmaceutical companies are testing and developing new drugs, and new drug delivery systems. For the first time, there is real hope for a cure.

A part of me also realizes, however, that it ultimately doesn't matter. We can all habituate to the sound. And when the sound stops bothering us, it's no longer a problem. At the end of the day, the truth is we don't need a cure, at least not to be healthy, happy, and productive members of society. The solution already exists inside each and every one of us.

From time to time, I still do struggle with my tinnitus, but never like I used to. If it spikes now, a few minutes of tinnitus meditation is all I need to find relief. It's a far cry from the endless agony I once had to endure.

No matter where you are with your tinnitus, no matter what setbacks or adversities you might face on your journey, you can start taking the steps to habituate. Even baby steps will get you there eventually. You can learn to live with this crazy condition and find the relief you so desperately deserve.

I wish you the best of luck on your journey, and above all else, remember: There is so much hope. You can, and you will, habituate to the sound of your tinnitus.

# Resources

### Rewiring Tinnitus Book Resources:

Rewiringtinnitus.com/bookresources

An up-to-date listing of all the important links and resources found throughout this book.

### The Tinnitus Relief Project:

Rewiringtinnitus.com/relief

A comprehensive set of brainwave entrainment audio tracks engineered to help you habituate to the sound of your tinnitus. Includes sound masking tracks, guided meditations, relaxation audio, focus enhancing tracks, and sleep induction music.

### The Rewiring Tinnitus Blog:

Rewiringtinnitus.com

The homepage of the Rewiring Tinnitus blog. I regularly post new articles, videos, tools and more. Sign up for the Rewiring Tinnitus newsletter to stay up to date with all of my work.

**The Rewiring Tinnitus Trigger Tool:**

Rewiringtinnitus.com/Journal

A fillable, 1-page, PDF tool that I created to help you track your lifestyle and discover what triggers your tinnitus and causes your tinnitus to spike.

**The Rewiring Tinnitus Facebook Page:**

Facebook.com/rewiringtinnitus

I post all my new articles and videos, as well as news and research from across the tinnitus community. Click "Like" to follow along.

**The American Tinnitus Association:**

ATA.org

The ATA is a US based nonprofit whose mission is to improve the lives of people with tinnitus and hyperacusis by providing hope of a quieter future through education, advocacy, and research toward a cure.

**The Vestibular Disorders Association:**

Vestibular.org

The Vestibular Disorders Association is an incredible nonprofit organization that goes above and beyond for the tinnitus community on a regular basis. For more than three decades, VEDA has been a highly respected source of scientifically credible information on tinnitus and vestibular disorders. Through their publications and online community, VEDA has reached millions of vestibular patients with critical information and support.

### Hearing Health Foundation:

HHF.org

Hearing Health Foundation is a wonderful U.S. based nonprofit organization with a mission to prevent and cure hearing loss and tinnitus through groundbreaking research and to promote hearing health through their free quarterly magazine. As the largest non-profit funder of hearing and balance research in the U.S., they have awarded millions of dollars to promising research initiatives, in areas such as hearing loss, tinnitus and hyperacusis.

### The British Tinnitus Association:

Tinnitus.org.uk

The British Tinnitus Association is a UK based nonprofit organization that strives to be the primary source of support and information for people with tinnitus and their careers in the UK and to advocate on their behalf. They aim to encourage prevention through educational programs and seek out effective management of tinnitus through their medical research program.

**Canadian Tinnitus Foundation:**

Findthecurenow.org

The Canadian Tinnitus Foundation is a not-for-profit organization dedicated to expanding awareness of tinnitus in Canada and generating funding for research to find a cure. Their mission is to provide a loud voice to those who suffer silently at the hands of this debilitating condition.

**The Tinnitus Research Initiative:**

Tinnitusresearch.org

The Tinnitus Research Initiative is a non-profit foundation dedicated to improving the quality of life for patients who suffer from tinnitus and related disorders. They believe that by bringing together researchers from a wide range of different disciplines, we will better understand tinnitus, leading to more effective treatments.

**Tinnitus Hub:**

Tinnitushub.com

Tinnitus Hub is a social enterprise dedicated to informing and educating the tinnitus community while offering safe self-treatment solutions. They provide unique services and tools to promote tinnitus knowledge and awareness, offer support for tinnitus sufferers, and raise funds for existing charities in the search for a cure. They also run the Tinnitus Talk support forum.

**Healthy Hearing:**

Healthyhearing.com

Healthy Hearing is an organization with a mission to educate about hearing loss and its implications. They connect people who need hearing help with qualified hearing care professionals with their online directory of consumer-reviewed clinics across the U.S. Healthy Hearing is the leading online information resource for hearing healthcare consumers and strive to provide unbiased, easy-to-understand content that is useful to our millions of visitors.

# Support Groups

**American Tinnitus Association Support Group Directory:**
ATA.org/managing-your-tinnitus/support-network/support-group-listing

**British Tinnitus Association Support Group Directory:**
Tinnitus.org.uk/directory

# Support Group Forums

**Tinnitus Talk:**
Tinnitustalk.com
Tinnitus talk is the largest online tinnitus support forum by far. With over 15,000 members, questions are typically answered quickly and by a large number of people. There are dozens of discussion boards covering everything from new research and clinical trials to treatments, alternative therapies, and general support. It's a wonderful place to learn more about tinnitus and talk to fellow patients.

**Tinnitus Sub-Reddit:**
Reddit.com/r/tinnitus
Reddit is essentially a website where anyone can set up a discussion board, called a sub-Reddit for any topic

they like. The tinnitus sub-Reddit is a highly active support group forum with several thousand members.

# Facebook Support Groups

**Tinnitus Sufferers:**
Facebook.com/groups/TinnitusSufferers/

**Living with Tinnitus and Hearing Loss:**
Facebook.com/groups/TinnituSupport/
**Hyperacusis and Tinnitus Support:**
Facebook.com/groups/233630540131144/

# Leave a Review!

Thank you so much for reading! I hope you've learned a lot.

Self-publishing this book was very much a labor of love. If you enjoyed reading it as much as I enjoyed writing it, or if you feel as though you've gotten something out of it, please take a minute and leave a review on Amazon.com!

Reviews help self-published authors like me to reach a wider audience, and in this case, that means helping more tinnitus sufferers around the world.

Thanks!

# Interested in One-on-One tinnitus coaching?

If you would like to learn more and work with me one-on-one, I've made it easy to get in touch! Simply visit Rewiringtinnitus.com/coaching or email me at Glenn@rewiringtinnitus.com.

I can offer a personalized strategy and approach to help you on your tinnitus journey.

# Works Cited

Bray, Roger. I Can Live With My Tinnitus: A Survival Guide For Tinnitus Sufferers. Self-published, 2016.

Harris, Dan. 10% Happier: How I Tamed the Voice in My Head, Reduced Stress Without Losing My Edge, and Found Self-Help That Actually Works-- A True Story. New York: Dey Street Books, 2014.

Hill, Julian Cowan. A Positive Tinnitus Story: How I Let Go of Tinnitus the Natural Way. Self-Published, 2014.

Salzberg, Sharon. *Lovingkindness: The Revolutionary Art of Happiness*. Massachusetts: Shambhala, 1995.

Schweitzer, Glenn. Mind Over Meniere's: How I Conquered Meniere's Disease and Learned to Thrive. Self-Published, 2015.

Stevenson, Shawn. Sleep Smarter: 21 Proven Tips to Sleep Your Way to a Better Body, Better Health and Bigger Success. Pennsylvania: Rodale, 2016.

# References

Baizer, Joan S, Senthilvelan Manohar, Nicholas A Paolone, Nadav Weinstock, and Richard J Salvi. "Understanding tinnitus: the dorsal cochlear nucleus, organization and plasticity." *Brain Research*, vol. 1485, 2012, pp. 40-53.

David, J Ben, Anthony Naftali, and Arie Katz. "Tinntrain: A multifactorial treatment for tinnitus using binaural beats." *The Hearing Journal*, vol. 63, no. 11, 2010, pp. 25-26, 28.

"Hearing Loss and Headphones - Is Anyone Listening?" *American Osteopathic Association*, www.osteopathic.org/osteopathic-health/about-your-health/health-conditions-library/general-health/Pages/headphone-safety.aspx.

Heller, Morris F, and Moe Bergman. "Tinnitus aurium in normally hearing persons." *Annals of Otology, Rhinology & Laryngology*, vol. 62, no. 1, pp. 73-83.

Margo, Jill. "Brain Changes Caused by Hearing Loss Can Be Slowed." *Australian Financial Review*, 4 Apr. 2016, www.afr.com/lifestyle/health/mens-

health/creeping-brain-changes-caused-by-
hearing-loss-can-be-slowed-20160404-gnxku3.

Morizono, Tetsuo, Michael M Paparella, and Steven K
Juhn. "Ototoxicity of Propylene Glycol in
Experimental Animals." *American Journal of*
Otolaryngology, vol. 1, no. 5, 1980, pp. 393-399.

Murata, Tetsuhito, Yoshifumi Koshino, Masao Omori,
Ichiro Murata, Masashi Nishio, Kazumasa
Sakamoto, Tan Horie, and Kiminori Isaki.
"Quantitative EEG Study on Zen Meditation
(Zazen)." *Psychiatry and Clinical Neurosciences*,
vol. 48, no. 4, 1994, pp. 881-890.

"Noise-Induced Hearing Loss." *National Institute on
Deafness and Other Communication Disorders*,
National Institute of Health, May 2015,
www.nidcd.nih.gov/health/noise-induced-
hearing-loss.

Shargorodsky, Josef, Sharon G Curhan, and Gary C
Curhan. "Change in Prevalence of Hearing Loss in
US Adolescents." *JAMA: The Journal of the
American Medical Association*, vol. 304, no. 7,
2010, pp. 772-778

# About the Author

Glenn Schweitzer is a small business owner, entrepreneur, and the creator of the popular Mind over Meniere's and Rewiring Tinnitus Blogs. He is passionate about helping others who suffer from tinnitus and vestibular disorders, and volunteers as an Ambassador Board Member for the Vestibular Disorders Association (VEDA). His works have been read by hundreds of thousands of tinnitus and Meniere's disease sufferers in over 160 countries worldwide. He continues to raise awareness for tinnitus, Meniere's disease, and other vestibular disorders, spreading his message of hope to those in need.

Feel free to contact Glenn at:
Glenn@Rewiringtinnitus.com

Made in the USA
San Bernardino, CA
01 September 2017